PHOTOGRAPHS BY JAKE WALTERS

HONEST

SALI HUGHES

FOURTH ESTATE · London

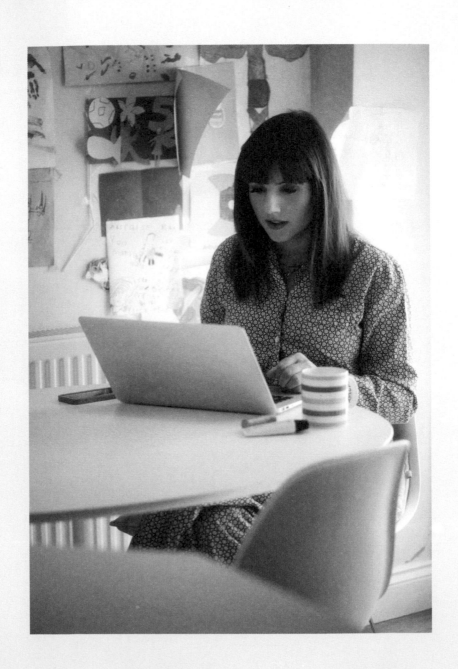

INTRODUCTION

'Pretty is something you're born with. But
beautiful, that's an equal opportunity adjective.'
Ralph Waldo Emerson

There are two mantras I live by. The first is my grandmother's. One day, as a very little girl, I sat on her bed watching her spritz on Yardley English Lavender perfume, powder her face from a gilt Stratton compact and slick on her fuchsia No7 lipstick. Transfixed, I asked her why she wore make-up. Clicking the lipstick shut she said, matter-of-factly, 'Because when I've got my make-up on, I'm always ready. Imagine if I was out and got some lovely invitation that I couldn't accept because I wasn't looking and feeling my best? With make-up, I'm always able to go on the adventure.' I never forgot it and I apply the same theory to most days. The other is one that I remind my friends of whenever they're feeling ill or blue, and I invariably send them a huge care parcel of beauty products and make-up. I believe that the only thing worse than feeling like crap, is looking like crap too. Often we can't do anything about the former, but I feel passionately that addressing the latter can only help.

I believe looking good to be an important and valid pursuit. All too often, women with an interest in their appearance are assumed to be stupid, shallow or unintelligent. Even traitors to feminism. But I see good grooming and feminism as entirely complementary. For some, beauty is a matter of pride and self-respect, of feeling your best and worthy of attention. While a man with an interest in football, wine, Formula 1 or even paintballing would never see his intelligence called into question, a woman with an interest in surface is perceived to have no depth. I believe it's perfectly normal to love both lipstick and literature, to be a woman who paints her nails while shouting at *Question Time*. Looking good makes us feel good, and the rituals involved are a pleasure in themselves. The implication that us poor women are getting up half an hour earlier than we want to and miserably trowelling on slap because it's what society tells us to do is absurd. I know categorically that for very many women, putting on make-up is the one and only time they enjoy to themselves all day. It's an act of love, self-care and, crucially, self-expression. Make-up is such a powerful tool of creativity. I genuinely pity men for not having it.

People often ask me, 'Why do you feel the need to put on make-up? Don't you love yourself without it?' It's a rather offensive and highly patronising question but one that, as a beauty columnist, I sadly come across every single day (primarily from people who seem to believe that washing their face in carbolic soap and cleaning their teeth with twigs makes them a much better and more intelligent person than me, obviously). The truth is, I go bare-faced constantly and my self-esteem is resolutely intact, thanks. But I would be miserable if I looked like that all the time. To me, deciding to be vampy one day, classic ingénue the next, painted Madonna on a Saturday night and bare-faced Joni Mitchell on a Sunday morning, is exactly what feminism is about: freedom.

And it has little to do with men (not that there's anything wrong with pulling make-up, frankly. We all like a jump, for heaven's sake). I wear make-up chiefly for myself, and apart from making me look better (I don't care who you are, everyone is improved by a little concealer and blush) and giving me confidence, it makes me happy.

Anyone who dismisses beauty and make-up as mere frippery, an irrelevance pursued by the vain, frankly knows nothing about women. During the best of times, we put on our face like armour, ready for whatever the day ahead throws at us. A slash of good lipstick has the power to make us feel more prepared for a big work presentation, a good base makes us more dynamic and ready to communicate confidently with others. I rarely even sit down and write in my pyjamas at home without a little tinted moisturiser and lip balm. Make-up, however subtle, provides the demarcation that the day has begun, and looking good bolsters us to get the hell on with it.

But for many women, looks become especially important at a time you'd perhaps least expect. During the darkest periods, beauty takes on an extra significance and, for many, can become one of our most effective coping mechanisms. When we've lost a job, are going through divorce, are grieving a loved one (I remember spending an hour or two choosing which lipstick to wear to my father's funeral. It seemed like the only thing I could control on such a tragic and unwanted day), we literally paint on a brave face. Even in economic crisis, we turn to beauty. Statistics consistently show that during times of recession and austerity, the sales of lipstick go up, due to the instant feel-good factor of buying and wearing a nice lippy. This lifting effect is perhaps never more utilised than during times of illness, when either the condition or its treatment has dramatically altered our appearance. Beauty rituals can become so much more than simple grooming – they can become a therapy in themselves.

To say I love beauty would be an understatement. I adore and revere it. Nothing makes me happier than discovering an amazing product and spreading the love, or popping into Selfridges for a Chanel lipstick on a rainy day, or mastering some technique I thought I'd never nail, knowing I can now rush off and share it with my friends. I've always been the same. From the moment I bought my first Body Shop Morello Cherry lip balm, I was hopelessly hooked. Within weeks, I was drooling over the 'Clinique Directory', a black and white catalogue of products, and binging on *Just Seventeen* beauty pages like some dirty junkie. I try several hundred products a year, across all price ranges, and my dining room resembles a small regional branch of Boots. I obsess over other women's routines, putting together bespoke goodie bags and performing makeovers whenever I'm allowed.

But there's a difference between being a beauty fan and someone who was born yesterday. Packaging and glossy ad campaigns sell pipe dreams and make promises that simply can't be kept. Myths are perpetuated and need to be broken. We spend our hard-earned money in billions on this stuff – shouldn't we know that what we're getting will work? I have spent 20 years, first as a make-up artist and then as a journalist, testing literally thousands of beauty products. I never recommend anything I haven't personally tried on myself, or on someone I know well. There is nothing more satisfying to me than looking at someone's beauty kit and letting her know she simply doesn't need the £80 eye cream, that the £25 moisturiser will work much better, that one concealer swapped for another will make her look fabulous in photographs in a way she never imagined, or that a new way of using cleanser will fix a lifetime of skin problems. I know what works and what doesn't and I want you to know too.

When I took over as beauty columnist on *Guardian* Weekend, I was determined to write a new kind of beauty coverage. I wanted to speak as freely as I do to my thousands of forum members and Twitter followers who ask me every single day for beauty advice and product recommendations. Glossy magazines, although I adore them more than most, and their often excellent beauty editors, simply cannot be wholly honest with you about beauty. They are at the mercy of major beauty advertisers, relying on them to keep them in business. If a major brand releases a moisturiser, a good write up is a dead cert. The problem is that while they will sometimes deserve them, there will be other occasions when a brilliant product from a smaller company, which doesn't have the same advertising spend, will have no chance of getting noticed. I'm here to make sure you don't miss out. I also want you to know the insider tricks I've learned from so many years working with the pros. Those looks you write to me about every single day are much simpler than you imagine. Smoky eyes, better-than-Botox make-up, winged liner, salon-precision nail painting? I have foolproof tricks for these and a hundred others that you'll use for the rest of your life.

I strongly believe that all women, without exception, look better with beauty products. Not a Jordanesque faceful, or pillowy cheeks stuffed full of fillers, but some – whether it's a little tinted moisturiser and mascara, or a swooshy eyeliner and red lips. And the key word here is 'better', because contrary to what the ad men want us to believe, I know that most women don't dream of having Cheryl Cole or Angelina Jolie's face. We don't look at supermodels and want to look like them, and live on cotton wool and Marlboro Lights. Overwhelmingly, we just want to look like ourselves, only *beautiful*. I'll help you do it.

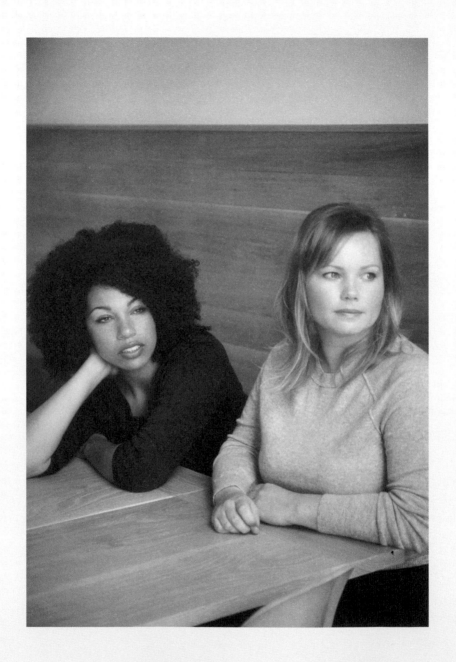

WHAT'S YOUR SKIN TYPE?

'I'm tired of all this nonsense about beauty
being only skin-deep. That's deep enough.
What do you want, an adorable pancreas?'
Jean Kerr

Ask anyone what is their skin type and most will say 'combination' or 'sensitive' – or both. Neither is as common as that. Women with a different answer will usually say 'dry', when in fact they are dehydrated. This must be overcome, because nothing in a bottle will improve your skin until you really know what you're dealing with. Arming yourself with your skin type, whether you are a textbook case of one, or a combination of 2–3 different types (menopausal women often find they run the gamut of skin types through the process of change), will allow you to buy the right products and stop wasting money on the wrong ones.

Skin typing is very useful, but of course not an exact science. It's perfectly possible to be 'a little from column A and a lot from column B'. For example, my skin is both dry and dehydrated but I find it responds best to products targeting the latter. My skin is rarely sensitive (miraculous, given how many products it endures in the name of research) but when it does flare up, cold weather and sugar are almost always at the scene. At which point, it is time to drop certain beloved products (those containing AHAs, for starters) temporarily from my routine. I know mineral oil sometimes makes me break out, but shea butter doesn't (it often does others). I know that a serum without the inclusion of hyaluronic acid will do nothing for me, but a facial oil without it will. This methodical thinking comes from knowing my own skin and observing it closely when times are good and bad. Skin typing is not a prescriptive business, it's really to help *you* to become an expert in your own skin, being aware of what your face loves and loathes and recognising when you can help and how.

Skin really is the beginning and end of beauty. With a canvas of great-looking skin, it's pretty hard to go wrong thereafter. And unlike make-up, hair and nails, skin is about so much more than appearance. It's your body's largest organ and the only one able to give you a daily visual update of its general health. Take advantage of that and listen to what it's telling you.

DRY

Feels uncomfortable and desperate for moisturiser
after cleansing or showering

....

Feels dry by the end of the day after proper
moisturising in the morning. Make-up is patchy

....

Feels sore in cold weather but is aggravated by central heating

....

Shows fine lines earlier than others in your peer group

....

Prone to dullness and flakiness, especially in winter
and around the nose, eyelids and cheeks

....

Feels dry when you wake up each morning without
a rich night cream before bed

....

Small pores

....

Prone to milia, the little white lumps that can hang around
for months, especially surrounding the eyes

I find women are increasingly calling themselves 'really dry'. I see this as a bit like wheat intolerance or Seasonal Affective Disorder – all are real, none are anything like as common as we're led to believe. Some dryness is usual but, mercifully, many of us haven't the faintest idea what it really means to be a genuine dry skin sufferer. Those with truly dry skin couldn't contemplate leaving the bathroom for breakfast without first applying rich moisturiser (my skin is so dry that I have to clean my teeth before showering – there's not enough time after exiting the shower to do so as by then my skin is so uncomfortable I have to grab some oil and cream immediately).

While summer generally offers some relief for sufferers, winter can be hell, and demands an extra emollient, take-no-prisoners, mega-moisturiser to avoid stinging, chapping, dullness and discomfort. Pharmacy and prescription brands like E45, Vaseline and Diprobase are often great on the body but can cause breakouts on the face (contrary to popular belief, dry skin can easily break out with trigger ingredients like mineral oil) and are very poor as a make-up base, which for me is almost as intolerable a predicament as the dryness itself. I'm of the opinion that the best treatment for a dry complexion – from slightly dry to parched and sore – involves the daily use of oily, soothing cleansing balms, high-grade plant oils, rich cosseting creams and gentle exfoliants.

SENSITIVE

Sometimes feels hot and itchy after cleansing

....

Flares up easily after using new skincare

....

Is more irritated at certain times in the menstrual cycle

....

Can be oily, combination, dry, dehydrated

....

Can come and go

....

Is prone to hot, itchy red blotches that get worse if touched

....

Sometimes angry-looking after a shower

....

Burns fast in the sun

Sensitivity is really bloody annoying if you love beauty. Lots of products contain active ingredients which, though perfectly safe, aggravate the skin of certain women to the point where they are either unpleasant or impossible to use. The problem is that very often women who believe themselves to be sensitive are actually only sensitive to one or two ingredients that are so prevalent in mainstream cosmetics that they seem impossible to avoid. Nonetheless, it's well worth working out what's causing the irritation. You need to do this through the rather tedious process of elimination: scaling your skincare right back then re-introducing each product one by one until you identify the offender. Fortunately, you may only have to do this once or twice in your life because a proper scan of a product's ingredient list may give you a good idea of what's causing the problem. You can then avoid it more easily because increasingly niche brands are ditching common irritants – mineral/palm/paraffin oils, fragrance, parabens, alcohol and so on (lots of people are perfectly fine to use these). It may occasionally mean paying a little extra, but this also seems to be changing. You can now buy decent non-irritating skincare in most high-street chemists and health-food shops. Sensitive types should also check their diets. Many experts will tell you there's no link between diet and skin but nothing will change my mind – I have known too many women, including myself, who see increased sensitivity when consuming too much sugar, and a significant decrease when we have a word with ourselves and stop. I am a decidedly orthodox person, I am big on chemicals and pretty sceptical on alternative therapies, but this is one area in which I believe in 20 years' client experience over science.

COMBINATION

Pores are larger around the nose, forehead and chin

....

Cheeks are generally normal, but prone to mild to moderate dryness

....

The T-zone: forehead, nose and chin are more oily and
spot prone, especially at certain times in the menstrual cycle,
during pregnancy or menopause

Most women I meet believe they have combination skin to some degree or another and I certainly agree that the majority of us will experience it at some point in our lives.

Combination skins are typically more likely to be sent off-kilter by hormones (period-related breakouts are common in combo types) and are particularly exacerbated by menopause. Sensible skincare is very important; I find that very often combination skin actually started out as relatively balanced skin that suffered ill treatment from either very harsh oil-stripping or inappropriately rich moisturising. Subsequently, the main goal is to not exacerbate either problem (forcing skin to opt for either extreme), so gentle, sympathetic skincare is essential. Most combination types prefer the texture, feel and staying power of oil-free moisturiser by day. This is fine, but I advise using balancing plant oils in the evening and regular use of a mild liquid exfoliant. I would counsel against the use of a foaming face wash particularly those containing sulphates (SLS). A balm, oil or cream cleanser is more sympathetic to unbalanced skins.

OILY

Shiny

....

Pores are large and easily visible (often with blackheads)

....

Prone to spots and / or acne (easily affected by hormones)

....

Ages more slowly, with fewer fine lines than others in your peer group

Comfortable upon leaving the shower, or after cleansing
(one could happily wander off for a cup of tea without craving moisturiser)

....

A single-ply tissue pressed to the chin and nose an hour after cleansing
will show translucent patches of oil

Oily skin is a double-edged sword and probably the trickiest and most unpredictable skin to treat. Double-edged, because it can make you quite miserable in your youth and even middle age (I see more older oily skins than ever), repaying you somewhat later by ageing more slowly overall. Dry skins enjoy greater clarity in youth but wrinkle more quickly as you age. Oily skin is tricky to treat, partly because of the skin itself but also because there is so much utter guff spoken about this type of skin that those who have it don't know what to do for the best. Oily skin can provide a short-term base for make-up, sending it packing almost as soon as it's landed, re-surfacing it with shine. (See the chapter on acne for the best way to care for oily, spot-prone skin.)

In summary, moisturisers and oils are certainly not to be avoided, but mineral oils are, shea and cocoa butters are, super-rich emollients are. I feel sad and frustrated by how many women have been convinced they must avoid oil to prevent oiliness. I am entirely understanding about why oil-free moisturisers are a more comfortable, matte and practical make-up base by day, but I would still advocate a light facial oil at night. It is simply not true that all oils are created equal. A good one will help oily skin, not harm it. Along with a gentle cleanser, it is your oily skin's best friend.

NORMAL

Neither oily nor dry (but occasional shine and dryness)

....

Comfortable, smooth

....

Small pores

I'm generally not a fan of the word 'normal' when applied to anyone's appearance but in this case, normal means well balanced – a skin that is neither dry nor oily, rarely a confused combination of the two. It hardly ever breaks out and mostly feels comfortable. If this is your skin, accept my congratulations. Your skin will be easy to manage and relatively forgiving during the ageing process. It may, at various times of the month or your life, temporarily wander into oily/combination/dry territory, at which point, you can adjust to more specific but mild products until it returns to normal. A little dryness during cold weather is to be expected in normal skin, as is mild oiliness and slightly larger pores in the T-zone, but this is rarely problematic. Don't go nuts and try to blitz momentary lapses in your otherwise great skin – over-zealous treatment of oiliness or dryness may endanger your usually normal state long-term.

DEHYDRATED

Prone to dullness, often lacklustre in appearance

....

Fine lines, some of which seem to come and go

....

Pinker (Caucasian) / brighter (Afro-Caribbean and Asian), plumper and healthier-looking immediately after showering (but before drying)

....

Responds positively to steam rooms, looks and feels better in humid weather conditions

....

Feels desperate for product after showering

....

Sometimes flakes and peels when make-up is applied, especially around the eyes and nose

....

Dry-feeling lips

Until quite recently, dehydration has been hugely conflated with dryness by the beauty industry, when in fact they are not the same thing at all. Dry skin lacks oil. Dehydrated skin lacks water (which is why dehydrated skins can easily be oily, not just dry). Dehydrated skin typically looks ten times better when soaking wet, then dull and drab when dried off with a towel. It comes alive in humid weather and looks grey in the cold. Some skins retain water better than others – there's no scientific proof that drinking water makes skin more moist, though there's a great deal of anecdotal evidence (most women I meet feel their skin looks better when they are drinking plenty of water). A senior dermatologist once told me, rather plausibly, that the body prioritises water consumption, allocating it first to vital organs. When the body becomes dehydrated, it will steal water from the skin, where it's less important. This makes complete sense to me, though true dehydration is obviously not the same thing as drinking two glasses of water per day, instead of eight.

What we do know is helpful to dehydrated skin are humectant ingredients that bind water to the surface. Glycerin (an oldie but a goodie) and hyaluronic acid are brilliant for this and agree with the vast majority of skins. I can't remember the last time I really loved a moisturiser that didn't include hyaluronic acid, it is truly miraculous at re-plumping the skin and imparting a nice, healthy-looking glow that is otherwise lacking in dehydrated skin. As one of the skincare ingredients we know absolutely does the job, it's becoming an increasingly common addition to products, from high end to mass market. Look out for it – it will make all the difference.

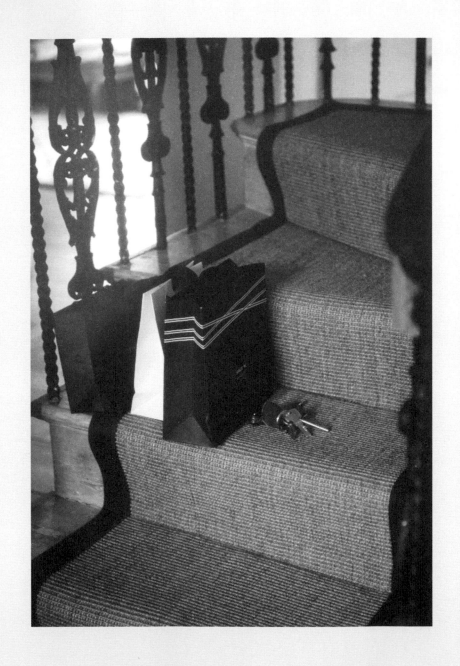

MANAGING COUNTER STAFF

'The most beautiful make-up of a woman is
passion. But cosmetics are easier to buy.'
Yves Saint Laurent

As a terrible truant (and, ultimately, a school drop-out), I was already to be found scoping out late-eighties department-store beauty counters at a very young age. The Clinique counter at Cardiff Debenhams was my most regular haunt and, like some sort of masochist, I visited regularly in my school uniform, knowing full well that I would at best be ignored and at worst humiliated and insulted. The counter manager was a woman who I knew, even at 12 or 13, was far too made-up. She had stiff, lacquered, short, bleached hair like Dolph Lundgren and wore enough make-up to see a regional chemist through rationing. She was beyond rude. And yet still I fixated on that counter, saving all my pocket money and allowance for the privilege of shopping there, not wanting to upset her.

One day, with enough money to buy a loose powder (yes, loose powder on a twelve-year-old is utterly lunatic but it came with a silver retractable brush that made me swoon), I went to the counter hoping I might find her on lunch break (I always imagined her angrily eating a Ryvita and refusing to budge up in the canteen), but no such luck. I asked for the coveted powder and she glared at me before telling me my skin was 'too bad' for it and to try Boots as it was 'much cheaper'.

I went home powderless and wrote my first letter of complaint, to Clinique head office. I listed this woman's countless acts of extreme rudeness and stated that, although I was a child, I was a customer nonetheless and a big fan of the brand. Two weeks later, a jiffy bag plopped through the letterbox containing a then-inconceivably expensive full-sized tube of body lotion and a pale green Clinique letterhead typed with an elegant and suitably appalled apology.

I have never been scared of beauty counter staff since. But I'm absolutely amazed at how commonly my grown-up, successful, smart readers tell me they daren't even visit a premium brand counter for fear of insult, ridicule or humiliation. These women – strong and assertive in all walks of life – shrink to pupae in the face of a shop assistant. They either leave counters empty handed, feeling upset and ignored, or having been bullied into submission and spent £300 on things they'll never use. This has to stop.

There is something uniquely personal about poor treatment at a beauty counter. Firstly, and most significantly, any interaction at the counter is by definition in reference to your face. A stranger is studying yours, must make value judgements upon it (and may not always do so tactfully), and is making suggestions on how to improve your appearance. This is potentially very problematic, even in the most sensitive hands.

Secondly, beauty counter staff are dressed up and made up to the nines (most are required to by contract). They can, unwittingly and wholly unintentionally, appear superior and intimidating, especially when you're on your last weary legs after an afternoon traipsing round town with whiney kids and a husband who forlornly sits in the nearest chair as soon as he enters the store. Thirdly, beauty consultants used to be bloody awful. I will accept no debate. Certainly, there were exceptions, but I absolutely know that cosmetics companies have only really understood the major importance of store-level customer service in the last twenty or so years. They are right to. Be nice today to a teen looking for spot cream and she's yours for life. Make a woman feel beautiful and she'll be back to buy every time she needs cheering. The problem is that most women already bear the psychic scars of mistreatment at the hands of old-fashioned consultants.

Let me just say that I worked in retail for five years. Serving customers is an honourable and noble profession and I have nothing but respect and admiration for the vast majority of retail workers who try to do it well. It takes enormous patience, diplomacy, effort and hard graft, for pretty poor wages. I can honestly say that I loathe rude customers as much as I detest rude counter staff. Like everything in life, it's a question of manners on all sides.

Today, there are very many excellent counter staff across all brands, in all parts of the country. I've seen fabulous, professional-looking makeovers at MAC, Laura Mercier and Bobbi Brown counters, expertly achieved by staff members on less than a tenner an hour. I've seen women visit the Crème de la Mer counter imagining it to be a traumatic experience, then seen them leave looking like a million dollars (and slightly high on free champagne and Belgian chocolates). The counter manager at Clinique in Brighton Boots is so cheery, so enthusiastic and warm, that women shopping only for Tampax and toothpaste queue up just to be rung through her till. There's a woman at my local Chanel counter who sneakily stashes away the limited edition nail polishes for my friend, knowing that she'll be in to purchase as soon as she can afford to. These are the staff who love beauty like we do, understand its powers, know that we won't forget good service, and enable our delicious habit to the delirious point of overdose.

These consultants are to be cherished. Treat them well. Do not speak down to them or take advantage of their generosity with time and samples. Booking in for an hour-long free makeover during a busy period then huffing when she dares to put through another customer's lipstick is unreasonable. Asking for a small number of samples is fine, expecting them on tap is not. Understand that she is required to offer you more products than you want and it's perfectly fine to not take that personally and politely say no. She is trying to get through the day, keeping both her customers and her bosses happy.

But my God, for every five goodies, there's some monster in inch-thick American Tan foundation and drawn-on eyebrows just waiting to harsh your mellow. And when you come across her, I beg you to stand firm, know it's your hard-earned cash she's after and understand that everything is your call. Here are some good starting points.

VOTE WITH YOUR WALLET

Counter staff work on commission. If you're getting rude or sloppy service from one sales assistant, politely move on to another and don't feel afraid to explain why. Helpful staff are more deserving of your money.

CHECK THE RETURNS POLICY

Major brands like Estée Lauder and Clinique have a policy of returning any product that causes a reaction, via head office (not on counter, as these are concessions within someone else's store). If you have sensitive skin, it might be less aggro to shop with these brands than to risk a frustrating refund row elsewhere.

COMPLAIN

Most companies are horrified when they hear of poor service and they should fix any issues (at 20 quid a lipstick, they can afford some extra staff training). The head office address will normally be on the back of a package and on the company website. Send a polite, serious letter with the time, date and location (and receipt details if available) of your purchase to the customer services and public relations department. You will almost certainly receive an apology and the store will be contacted about the complaint.

BE FIRM

Easier said than done but it's time to man up. This is your face and your purse and you decide what happens to both. If a sales assistant starts trying to push you into buying things you don't want, don't panic and don't say you'll come back later. Just smile and say firmly, 'No, I am sure I have everything I want today, thank you' and leave.

WEAR A GOOD BAG

On one hand, everyone should be treated well, regardless of age or apparent wealth, but on a busy counter, the woman who looks like she can shop will always get preferential treatment. Even if you've dashed out in a onesie and mad hair, carry a decent bag. It won't go unnoticed and, miraculously, you'll suddenly find staff a whole lot more attentive.

ASK FOR SAMPLES

If you're not sure you want to buy a product a consultant is trying to sell you, ask for a sample. Most counters now have either pre-packed samples across the range or stacks of empty pots for decanting a small supply to try at home. Kiehl's, Clarins, Laura Mercier and Space NK are especially great for this. Don't abuse the privilege – two to three samples, perhaps more if you're buying something, seems fair to everyone.

DON'T BUY ACROSS-BRAND

I hate it when sales associates say you must buy a whole skincare range for it to work properly. This is usually balls and if it isn't, I always have grave reservations about any product that can't stand on its own two feet. If you love one brand, then go for it. But no two skincare products in my routine are alike. It's a question of playing to the strength of different companies (I'd buy primer from Laura Mercier, but foundation from Armani, for example). If they insist you need their moisturiser for their serum to work, walk away and get a better one.

KNOW HOW YOU WANT TO LOOK

It's your face and you know it far better than they do. If you tell them your skin is oily, they should listen. If you know your eyes are blue, they must not tell you they're green. If you want red lipstick, you must have it. If you have a maximum of thirty pounds to spend, then that is the limit. Do not let someone on commission tell you how to look. You know better, always.

BE SMART ABOUT MAKEOVERS

Do not book an on-counter makeover before an important event, unless you've been to that particular artist before and were happy with the result. I've seen some on-counter reader makeovers that were so hamfisted and clueless, they caused me actual bodily pain. Some brands are better than others. I find Bobbi Brown, MAC, Charlotte Tilbury, Laura Mercier, Illamasqua and Armani staff generally more reliable and skilful than those at other brands, but of course, there are many exceptions on both sides so don't bank on anything unless you have time to fix it afterwards. And please don't take advantage of consultants or deliberately mislead them. They're not idiots, can spot a freeloader a mile off and always, always know if you've popped in for a free makeover with zero intention of buying. I personally feel that a good free makeover deserves a lipstick purchase. That way, s/he gets a sale and you get to touch up her handiwork later on.

THINK BEFORE YOU SHARE

Don't give a sales associate your phone number, ever. No good can come of it. Find out what will happen if you surrender your email and whether it will remain exclusive to that counter. Sometimes alerts on in-store discounted beauty shopping events are useful; constant inbox spamming over everything from games consoles to breadmakers, not so much.

ADOPT A ZERO-TOLERANCE POLICY ON RUDENESS

If counter staff say anything that you wouldn't accept from a stranger in a call centre, or on the street, move on. It's your money and their job. If they want neither, screw them. Leave, calm down and pick it up with head office.

GIVE GOOD FEEDBACK

How can stores and brands know what they're doing right if you don't tell them? Positive feedback about a great member of on-counter staff will be gratefully received and cumulatively acted upon. Consultants with consistently great feedback move ahead and ultimately get their own counters, their own stores, their own regions. Play a part in the process of getting good service for everyone.

BAD BEAUTY COUNTER LEXICON: THE WORDS WE DREAD TO HEAR

'You're very pale – let's warm you up'
(make you as orange as me)

....

'If you buy two more things, you get two free gifts'
(an acid-green eyeshadow and a half-sized
lipstick the colour of an Elastoplast)

....

'Sorry, I don't normally work on
this counter so I don't know'
(I'm covering a lunchbreak and I can't
be arsed to earn someone else commission)

....

'This moisturiser is designed to be used in
conjunction with the matching eye cream,
which is designed to work with the co-ordinating
eye-lift serum, and so you need all three to
get the benefit' (this product is pants but I
get a bonus every time I sell the set)

....

'This will actually reverse the ageing
process of your skin' (you might as well
Google 'snake oil' and set fire to your wallet)

How to spot a brilliant consultant

S/he tells you when different brands make something better than hers. A consultant who says 'Our lipsticks are great, but if you're only going to own one blusher, make it a Nars' is a star. Trust her.

....

S/he tells you twice as many things that are lovely about your face than things you can improve. For example, 'Your skin is clear enough to only wear tinted moisturiser ... We could make your eyes seem bigger with pale shadow – you can wear shimmer as you don't have any lines there.' This is nice, professional and polite.

....

S/he looks good. I don't mean beautiful, I mean well presented. A woman who understands how to make the best of what she has, and knows what good hair and make-up actually looks like, is someone you can trust to do the same for you.

....

S/he asks questions. A good consultant won't give you a makeover or lesson without finding out how much time you have to get ready each day, how much make-up you already own, how advanced your existing skills are, how you actually want to look. People who love beauty are curious about beauty. They can't help themselves asking.

....

S/he is still nice to you when you don't buy anything. The clincher. A sales consultant who still makes you feel good about browsing will get the future sale, again and again.

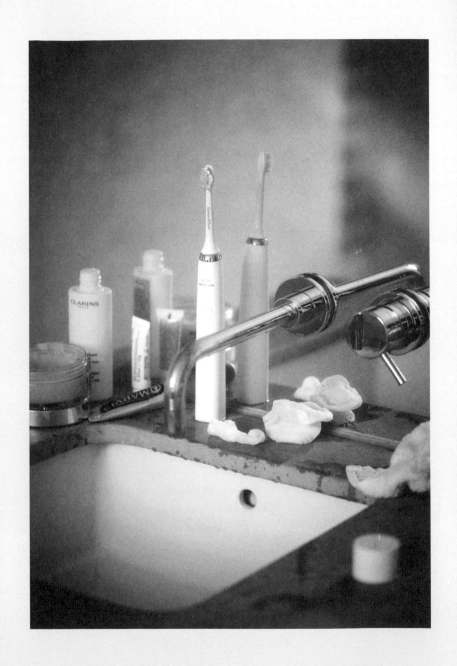

YOUR DAILY SKINCARE ROUTINE

'I have but this to say, sunburn is beauty suicide.'
Helena Rubinstein

Ask anyone, even now, how one best looks after skin and 90 per cent will either say 'soap and water' or 'cleanse, tone, moisturise' whether they themselves do it or not. Meanwhile, I look after my skin quite carefully – though certainly not obsessively – and even I couldn't entertain the 12-step cleansing rituals I read about on the internet. Who has the time? Frankly, who even has the skin? Theirs must be reinforced with carbon to withstand all that pummelling. But nor do I believe that soap and toner is going to pass muster. Skin is our largest organ and the only one on show to the world wherever we go. It deserves our respect and will respond very kindly to some daily attention. And yes, it really does need to be daily.

People find basic skin maintenance a drag but we are talking just a few minutes' work that absolutely will make you look better. You will get into the habit very quickly and the result will come fast. I also have little time and more pressing tasks to complete, so I skip what's not, in my opinion, wholly necessary. Toner, lovely though it may be, is almost entirely useless, and yet I'd sooner go without petrol than serum. Do you need to wear primer? Sometimes. Do you know when in your routine you're supposed to apply it? Possibly not. For me, the most important steps in caring for your skin are to cleanse, treat, moisturise and protect. I do this with cleanser, serum, moisturiser and sun protection. The whole thing takes me five minutes. The rest is mere details. Here's how it breaks down.

1. Cleanse

Why?

I bang on about this, but removing make-up and dirt through proper cleansing is absolutely essential. And not with wipes – the beauty equivalent of cleaning your clothes in air freshener. Wipes are for use only in extremis (or, as my friend Caroline Hirons so brilliantly puts it, purely for 'Flying, festivals and fannies' – I would only add 'falling down drunk'). When I say cleanse, I mean with a cream, balm or oil, though I'm not keen on the latter as they require a separate eye make-up remover and, also, I find the trickles down my pyjama sleeves extremely annoying. I'm also not keen on facial washes, since they rarely remove every trace of make-up (I find faint foundation stains on the towel) and often contain sulphates to make them foam.

In any case, brand and price here is not wildly important, what is more crucial is that you use whatever product you buy, though in general, I would recommend you avoid cleansers containing mineral oils if you're spot-prone (there are some notable exceptions – Eve Lom's cleanser is mineral-oil based and I've seen it work wonders on some problem skins). Secondly, you will need a flannel / face cloth of the old-fashioned terry cotton variety – the kind your gran used or which you might steal from a hotel. Many modern cleansers come with a muslin cloth; by and large, these are not the best thing for the job. Unless you have very sensitive skin, weeping acne pustules or rosacea, a flannel is much better. Save the muslins for cleaning up dinner from the kids' faces. The flannel is important here because it removes the cleanser and gunk beneath very effectively and at the same time buffs away dead skin cells that cause blackheads and make the complexion appear flaky, dull and dry.

When?

Twice a day, morning and night. I do my morning cleanse before stepping into the shower and my nighttime cleanse before bed. If you get very sleepy and lazy as the evening progresses, remove your make-up as soon as you get in from work, then you can relax. Whatever your chosen routine, just make sure you do it – I promise your skin will be transformed.

Method

Massage a large blob of cleansing cream or balm into your face, covering the eye area. Don't forget your forehead, neck and jawline. Don't be mimsy – you can be firm here. Soak the face cloth in hand-hot water and wring out. Place it over your face and press down gently for a few moments. Then wrap it around your hand like a mitt and buff off the cleanser in circular movements, starting with the eyes, then more firmly across the rest of the face. Rinse the cloth halfway through to get rid of the gunk. If your make-up is very heavy, repeat the whole process.

2. EXFOLIATE

Why?

This is an extra treatment and not one that needs doing every day. I exfoliate my skin with an AHA-based liquid a couple of times a week. The more spot-prone can ramp things up to once a day. The product you choose here is more important than before. BHAs (beta hydroxy acids, usually salicylic) are very effective on spot-prone skins. AHAs (alpha hydroxy acids, like glycolic, lactic and citric) have great anti-ageing properties and are commonly used in stronger concentrations in chemical peels. Liquid exfoliants are very effective in treating fine lines, enlarged pores, dullness and minor pigmentation marks and the difference after a short time of using them regularly is usually visible.

I appreciate acid is a word that sounds bloody scary in relation to beauty products, but don't be afraid. These are natural acids in over-the-beauty-counter dilutes and so simply aren't strong enough to do anything really drastic. They do, however, require some caution. You should always start with a mild formula and use only once in the first week. Avoid any that list alcohol as their first ingredient as these will almost always dry out your skin, which is no good (there are a couple of exceptions, including my favourite exfoliant, Liquid Gold. But it's more helpful in the first instance for you to hold back on the alcohol). See how your skin responds (some tingling is normal), then leave it for a couple of days.

Secondly, whether you are a seasoned exfoliator or a novice, it is absolutely essential that you follow up with sunblock (a broad-spectrum SPF of 30 or above) if going outside. Exfoliants work by gobbling up the dead upper cells, exposing virgin skin beneath. This new skin is more vulnerable to sun damage and needs protecting. This is why I always do any acid-exfoliation at nighttime and apply sun protection the next morning. If you have eczema, rosacea or extremely sensitive skin, you can skip this step altogether.

When?
Once a week for the first week, then, if there's no adverse reaction, two to three times a week thereafter.

Method
After cleansing, soak two cotton wool discs in liquid exfoliant. Sweep them over your entire face, including the neck and around the mouth. I also do my eye area as it can become flaky, but if your eyes are very sensitive, don't. Wait a few moments for the wetness to disappear (don't egg things on with a towel) before moving on to the next step.

3. SERUM

Why?
Serum is for addressing specific skin concerns and there are thousands of products available for each one. Some serums treat dehydration, others large pores and spots, some tackle wrinkles, some fade dark spots, others exfoliate. Some do two or more jobs under a banner term of anti-ageing. What they all have in common is a very fine texture that penetrates quickly into the upper layers of the skin. They are generally non-oily and broadly contain higher concentrates of key treatment ingredients than moisturisers. They usually don't contain enough moisture to be used alone and you'll need to follow up with a cream or oil for added comfort and protection.

When?
Every morning and night. You can use two different serums – one at each time of day – for two different skin conditions, or the same one, as desired. I use a hyaluronic acid-rich serum in the mornings to plump up my dehydrated skin and give a nice base for make-up. In the evening, I use a multi-purpose anti-ageing serum to treat fine lines, dullness and slackening.

Method
After cleansing (and exfoliating where applicable), place two to three drops of serum onto your fingertips and massage into the entire face and neck, including the eyes. Don't be feeble and stroky here, massage firmly but comfortably into the skin. Wait a few moments for any wetness to subside, then move on to the next step.

4. Moisturiser

DAY CREAM

Why?

Nowadays, most people agree that moisturiser is essentially A Good Thing. It makes skin feel more comfortable and supple, look plumper, brighter and better and shields it against the elements. It is not to be avoided, however oily and spot-prone your skin (see Acne for a full explanation on why this is not a good idea). I know for a fact that moisturiser improves the quality of the surface layer of skin. That is really good. But I don't believe it alters much below that, chiefly because it can't get down there. I'm not at all convinced that it can 'fix' any problems and I certainly don't believe it can alter the structure of the skin, I'm sorry to say. When I speak to women about their skin, I realise just how much cod science is fed to us all via packaging and advertising, until even the most intelligent reader believes that miracles come in a small expensive pot. Personally, I almost always choose day creams according to how they make my skin look and feel immediately upon application and how good a base they provide for make-up. I rarely consider their long-term benefit claims.

The other point of confusion is sun protection. Many day moisturisers include SPF (usually 15, sometimes 8, 12 or 30). I am broadly in favour of them, except that so many SPF moisturisers peel off in little balls when you try to apply make-up over them, which drives me to distraction and then straight to the sink to start all over again. SPF creams can also, very often, make eyes water, so you will probably need a separate eye cream. There's an argument that SPF moisturisers shouldn't be used as they'll stop your cream from properly sinking in and treating the skin. I personally disagree with this because a) I don't believe moisturisers can do this, sun protection or none; b) sun protection is important and I am realistic enough to know that if wearing it is time consuming and not easy, people simply won't do it.

You may want to choose a tinted moisturiser in place of a regular one, though they rarely provide enough moisture for this to be comfortable so I'd suggest layering them over a thin coating of day cream. It's your call. All I ask is that in autumn and winter you wear some form of broad-spectrum (protecting against both UVA and UVB) sun protection either via your day moisturiser, primer, foundation or BB cream. An SPF of 15 or above is fine – you won't be out very much and sunlight appears for a short time anyhow. Besides, vitamin D from the sun is important. In spring and summer, or in a sunny climate, you should start using a broad-spectrum sunblock of SPF 30+. You can either use this over moisturiser (a few minutes later), or alone over serum. Again, there's an argument for not doing this, but as someone with very dry skin myself, I know how much more comfortable and moist my skin feels in the summer months, and also how much more moisturising and sophisticated modern sunblocks are. And, most importantly, I want people to be able to easily protect their skin. Not enough people do.

When?
Every morning.

Method
After serum, warm a little day cream or lotion between your fingertips and massage into the skin using deep, firmish movements. Don't rub back and forth, especially if your day cream contains SPF, as this often causes it to disintegrate into little balls, which is maddening.

NIGHT CREAM OR FACIAL OIL

Why?
Because you've just cleansed and your skin needs moisturiser overnight. Your skin will feel more comfortable and look heaps better the following morning if you wear it – brighter, plumper, more awake. You will also be much less likely to have droopy crease marks when you wake up (silk pillowcases, available from beauty boutiques, also stop this happening). Whether you use cream or a plant oil in the evening is up to you. I almost always wear oil because I find it impractical during the daytime – make-up doesn't go especially well over the top of it. In either case, it's worth choosing a night moisturiser that's a bit richer than your day cream because you'll rub plenty off onto your pillowcase and because it doesn't matter if you're shiny when you're asleep, so you might as well treat yourself. I like to be able to still feel some tack from my night moisturiser when I touch my face in the morning. If I can't, I upscale to something heavier.

When?
Every night, after serum.

Method
For night cream, use the same application method as day cream (see above). For facial oil, warm a few drops in the palms of your hands and massage it into your face and neck, pressing firmly into the skin. You will need to avoid the eye area as oils can cause puffiness or, more seriously, a build up that can clog lash follicles and lead to blepharitis, an extremely uncomfortable and unsightly swelling and reddening of the eyelids (yes, I have been there. I don't recommend it). Creams can also clog lash follicles but it seems to be much less common.

Incidentally, if your skin is super dry and it feels nice to add night cream over the top of facial oil, i.e. to use both at the same time, then go for it (in that order). It's also perfectly fine to squeeze a few drops of plant oil onto your fingertips and mix it with your night cream before applying, to save time and hassle. I often do this myself in the winter or whenever I crave a moisture boost.

OPTIONAL EXTRAS

Eye make-up remover
If your cleansing balm is gentle and you use a flannel to remove it, then you won't need a separate eye make-up remover. I only ever really use them to make quick eye make-up changes and to correct smudges. Still, if you want to use it, bear in mind that you'll need an oil-based one to remove waterproof mascara. Otherwise, water-based is fine (and doesn't cause blurriness). Before cleansing, drench a cotton wool disc and sweep over the eyes, using a different disc on each eyelid.

Face masks
If you like applying face masks to boost skin hydration, treat spots or brighten your complexion, use them after cleansing but before serum, once or twice a week or whenever you need a boost. Follow the packaging instructions for application.

Toner
If you enjoy using toner, I'm all for it, but please don't use it just because someone on a counter or in a salon said you need it to 'remove the last traces of cleanser and close pores'. Neither of these things is true. Water via a cloth removes cleanser best, and toner cannot close pores. The only good reason to use these lovely but largely useless scented waters is because you love them. After cleansing but before serum, soak a cotton wool disc and sweep it all over, or pour it into a spritz bottle and mist it over your face.

Eye cream

See the chapter on basic kit for my views on eye cream. But essentially, if you experience no irritation or puffiness from using your everyday face moisturisers and anti-ageing products around the eye area, save your money and continue using them. If they aggravate – or if you use plant oil as a night cream – you'll need an eye cream. These are patted around the eye area with your ring finger, starting in the inner corner and moving outwards to the other side, then downwards towards the nose. Use after serum.

Spot treatments

If you have prominent spots, you'll probably want to treat them overnight. High-concentration salicylic gel works best. After the rest of your skincare routine is finished, dab the gel directly onto the spot with a clean cotton bud. Tingling is normal.

Primer

Primer isn't really skincare, it's a silicone balm designed to give a smooth and long-lasting base for make-up. There's more on primer in the chapter on foundation, but if you decide to use it, primer goes on after all your other skincare, as the last step before make-up. I wouldn't in all honesty use primer if you are also wearing sunblock, simply because it feels like playing Buckaroo with your face – there's only so much you can lay on it and still have things work. Smooth primer on without rubbing and leave it for a few moments to set.

Skincare crib sheet: what goes on in which order

Morning

Cleanser

....

Toner (optional, wholly unnecessary)

....

Serum

....

Eye cream (optional)

....

Day cream

....

Sunblock (if not otherwise protected)

....

*Primer (optional – I would generally only wear
it if not wearing sunblock)*

....

Make-up (optional)

EVENING

Eye make-up remover (if desired)

....

Cleanser

....

Exfoliant (2–3 times a week, not in conjunction with toner)

....

Serum

....

Eye cream (optional)

....

Oil / Night cream / Both

....

Spot treatment (optional)

1–2 TIMES A WEEK

Face mask (optional)

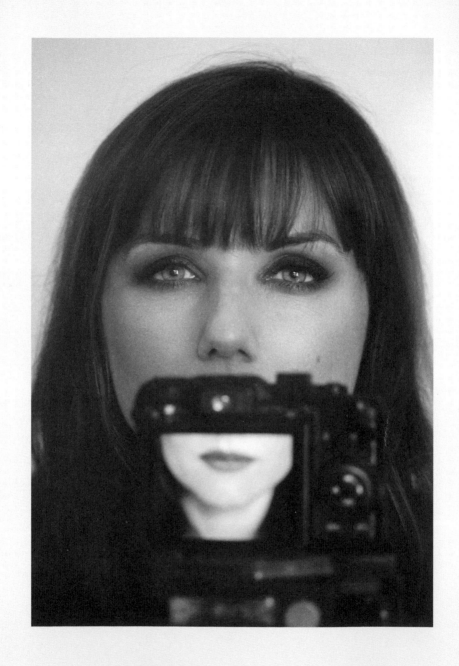

HOW TO LOOK GOOD IN A PICTURE

'They used to photograph Shirley Temple through gauze.
They should photograph me through linoleum.'
Tallulah Bankhead

When I was told my enlarged, largely unretouched, decidedly imperfect and un-model-like face would appear close-up in the paper every Saturday, I could have cried. It is a very strange thing to watch yourself ageing in eight-week blocks, despite knowing, after over two decades in the business, that photographs are largely unrepresentative of a person's face. I say this because it's a mistake to scrutinise your face in close-up and be under the illusion that this is how you look. In the flesh, other people glance at your face as a whole – a moving, changing image affected by different lights, words and facial expressions.

Three years later, I am pretty blasé about having my photograph taken. Truly, I've gone from being camera-phobic to reasonably photo-genic and believe me when I say that it's entirely learnt behaviour. And you don't need to be on a public stage to get there. You don't need to look like a Euro-bomber in your passport photo, and there are ways of posing for wedding photographs that don't make you hide the album in a lead box as soon as it arrives. There's good reason to overcome your fear of looking terrible on camera. One friend of mine almost always refused to have her photo taken, conscious of her weight and face. This is very common and extremely sad. She finally snapped out of it when her husband pointed out that if anything were to happen to her tomorrow, her refusal to pose for photographs would mean that her son had little to remember her by. This may sound morbid but it isn't only significant in death – by refusing to be photographed you are denying others, but most of all yourself, many happy memories.

That said, I am not suggesting you should strike some unnatural supermodel pose whenever a camera appears. Not at all. For the most part, we all should and do accept that we sometimes look crap in photos and don't much care – their function is to be a record of a lovely time, not to make us feel like Gisele. But there are some images that it is good to get right, not least because we have to see them frequently – such as office security passes and railcards, or long-term, such as wedding albums and passports. A daily glance at an unflattering photo is a downer and largely unnecessary if you know the tricks.

Make-up is a start, sure. Some products make you look as though you've been wearing skiing goggles in tropical sunlight as soon as a camera flash hits you, while some magically bathe you in flattering faux candlelight. But some poses sculpt the face in a way you never thought possible, while others guarantee nine chins. Here are my tricks to getting it right, but before you start, look at lots of pictures of yourself you like and try to work out why you like them – what's the common thread? Do you look better from one side of your face than another? Best when relaxed and laughing or more considered? Hair up or down? There will be something in common with every photograph of yourself that you love. Identify it. That's your starting point. For anything else, there's a quick fix.

COMMON PROBLEMS IN PHOTOGRAPHS – AND HOW TO FIX THEM

Problem
Two-tone face and neck. Whatever your natural colouring, you'll sometimes see in pictures that your face is white but your neck isn't – either it's much darker or, worse, ruddy. This is because flashlight bounces off the face but it is absorbed by the recessed neck and chest area. It creates the effect of appallingly matched foundation.
Fix
Avoid fake tan unless you are taking it over the entire face, and ensure your foundation is well matched (see the Foundation chapter). Dust a little illuminating face powder all over the neck and any exposed chest to catch the light and give a more uniform tone.

Problem
Grey, dull passport photo.
Fix
Firstly, for God's sake choose a digital photo booth where you can select the photo only when you're happy with it. Those old-style booths that spit out a revolting surprise are an expensive nightmare. Most stations

now have these newer versions. Alternatively, go to a photo shop. These usually offer a service where a photographer takes a passport photo against an approved background, using a normal camera on a tripod. The result is usually far more flattering and they will probably take several to choose from (they are also, in my experience, the only way to get a baby passport photo). In either case, take with you an A4 or A3 sheet of white paper and hold it a few inches under your chin. It will give a more flattering, brighter result and help minimise under-eye circles. When you're happy with a passport photo, you can avoid repeating the ordeal by scanning it to be reused for security passes, travelcards and so on.

Problem
White rings around the eyes.
Fix
I see this so often, I could weep. Unless you've recently returned from a fortnight in Val d'Isère, the blame here can be laid squarely at the door of the hugely popular light-reflector pens (YSL Touche Éclat, Clinique Airbrush Concealer and many, many more). These are great products but they should match the colour of your skin (most women seem to wear one that's far too pale and pink) and must be applied with some self-control. All too often, women plaster them on to conceal dark circles, but this is not their rightful job. Instead, cover dark circles with a concealer that has only mild light-reflective properties (Clarins, Nars and Clinique make excellent ones for all skin colours). If you want a little extra light, pat some light-reflector pen over the top, but go easy.

Problem
Stark white face (Caucasian), bluish face (Eastern Asian), ashy, ill-looking face (Asian, Caribbean, African).
Fix
This is often a sunblock problem. Mineral sunscreens contain zinc or mica, which has a naturally chalky finish. It gets much worse in flashlight. Sun protection is important, yes, but consider switching to a chemical sunscreen if nice photographs are important.

Problem
Double or triple chins.
Fix
Everyone has at one time or another gasped at the sight of their numerous chins in a photograph. Obviously weight and skin slackening are contributing factors but no one is wholly immune. Whatever the cause, poses and angles help a lot. Firstly, pose with the camera slightly above your face (looking down) never underneath you. Secondly, pop your tongue into the roof of your mouth. It will lift any extra skin underneath your chin. Models do it all the time and it works a treat.

Problem
Naff pout.
Fix
It is perfectly reasonable to want your lips to look fuller and sexier in a picture, but pouting, unless played for laughs, always looks obvious and silly. For a more subtle but effective way to add fullness, push your tongue against the inside of your top teeth – either smiling or not. Doing this pushes the jaw and the mouth outwards, and also gives cheekbones a bit of extra definition (that sucking in your cheeks thing looks mad). Try it, it totally works.

Problem
Squinting.
Fix
For some reason, this, in my experience, happens a lot to people with green or blue eyes. The camera flash of multiple photographs leaves the eyes almost unable to open completely, making for a squinty face in the final shot. When flash is relentless like this, close your eyes completely and try to relax them. Tell the photographer to count you down 3-2-1 to shot. Then open your eyes just as s/he takes the shot. Your eyes won't have time to take in the light and squint. I do this a lot on shoots.

Problem
Looking away.
Fix
It seems obvious but almost everyone instinctively looks at babies, friends, animals or anything else in the frame, rather than towards the camera. The ideal is to look into the lens, never towards the flash, as this causes red eye. And as with any important picture, take loads and loads. There's a safety in numbers – the more shots taken, the more chance there is of a great one being taken among them. And relax in the knowledge that, these days, anything can be deleted. For every shot in the *Guardian*, I've posed for around 30 (and I still moan about the one they pick).

Problem
Unnatural smile.
Fix
You have almost certainly been waiting too long for someone to press the damn button. Any smile looks fake and frozen after 30 seconds or so. Relax your face completely, move your jaw around – gurn if you have to. Then start again.

Problem
Drab skin.
Fix
Your problem here may be background. Green makes skin look awful, unless you're very red, in which case it can help tone things down. For the rest of us, grass is pretty unflattering (why are all wedding photos taken on lawns?) – stone, a painted wall, even pavement is much nicer against skin. White, black, cream and grey backgrounds always work – the plainer the better. Yellow can look very nice, and gold looks absolutely beautiful (photographers sometimes hold gold cardboard under a model's face for this reason).

Problem

Blank expression.

Fix

I've seen the most talented actors become dead-eyed the minute they step in front of a camera, their expressive faces instantly becoming blank. To avoid this, look at your feet and count to three. On three, look up at the camera (or ask the photographer to call your name). Your face will instinctively appear more expressive and interesting, as though you are thinking something. It looks much better.

MAKE-UP THAT LOOKS GREAT IN PHOTOGRAPHS

RED LIPSTICK

It makes teeth look whiter, skin clearer and provides a great focal point. Just make sure it's applied neatly and freshly, as any smudges and wobbles will show up.

CONCEALER

Everyone looks better with concealer, that is just a fact. Use it to cover dark circles, spots, uneven skin tone and broken veins. Choose one that's yellow-based. Nars, Bobbi Brown, Clinique, Kevyn Aucoin, Clarins and Armani make brilliant ones.

FACE POWDER

I love face powder and never more so than for photo shooting. It evens out skin tone and removes shine, giving pictures a more professional and smart quality. I use Bobbi Brown, MAC, Chantecaille or Nars.

EYELASH CURLERS

Nothing appears to open up your eyes like a great curler. Unfortunately, you do get what you pay for – I like those by Suqqu, Urban Decay, Shu Uemura and Kevyn Aucoin.

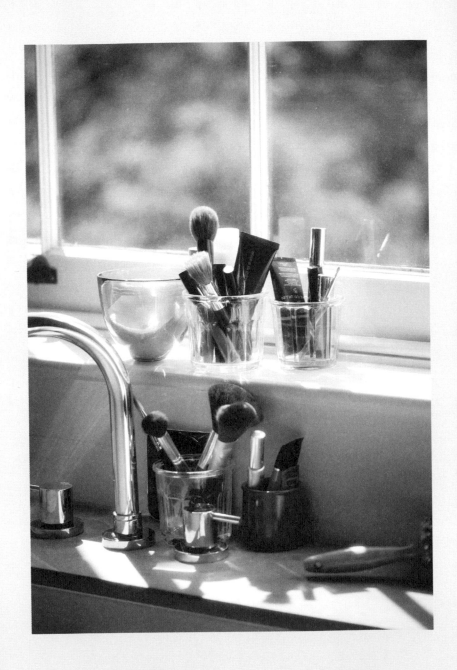

BASIC KIT:
THE PRODUCTS YOU NEED NOW
(AND THE STUFF YOU DON'T)

'Joy is the best make-up. But a little
lipstick is a close runner-up.'
Anne Lamott

I own thousands of beauty products. I love looking at them, playing with them and keeping abreast of what's new. But there are some items I never replace – a tinted moisturiser that erases the evidence of five vodkas the night before, the mascara that never migrates to my cheeks, the blusher that makes me look like I've just had amazing sex, the nappy ointment that hides the hallmarks of an enthusiastic snog beforehand. These are the things I am simply never without and would replace immediately if my luggage went missing at the airport. What's important here is not necessarily the product itself (your taste in brands, skin type and colouring will vary from mine), but the unique job it performs in my everyday life. Together, these tools make up my beauty arsenal and ensure that, whatever invitation pops up, I can always get ready.

CREAM OR BALM CLEANSER

It is practically impossible to have good skin long term without good cleansing. There are milks (great), washes (less good) and oils (good but too messy if wearing nice pyjamas), but a cream or balm cleanser will serve every one of every skin type very well. A decent one will remove every last trace of make-up and prepare your face for treatment products and a good night's sleep. I love those by Clarins, Aurelia, REN, Elemis, Weleda, Body Shop, Aromatherapy Associates, Liz Earle and Simple.

Massage into dry skin, including around the eyes, and remove with a hot, wrung-out flannel. Rinse the flannel and repeat the process if wearing very heavy make-up. Change your flannel each morning.

LIQUID EXFOLIANT

Not to be confused with a classic toner, which is basically lovely smelling water and wholly useless (if you love using it, go ahead. Just don't kid yourself it's actually doing anything that water isn't doing better). By contrast, a liquid exfoliant is a very useful product containing either AHAs or BHAs, which help to remove dead skin cells and refine pores. If you are someone with acne, buy a BHA liquid. If you are dull of complexion or just looking to minimise the appearance of lines and pores (very common in women over 35), invest in AHAs. Many liquid exfoliants combine both acid types, which can work well. I like liquid exfoliants by Clarins, Alpha H Liquid Gold, Pixi, Mario Badescu, Elizabeth Arden, REN and L'Occitane.

Every other day and after cleansing (every third day if sensitive), soak a cotton wool disc with the exfoliant and sweep it over the face. Allow to dry for a few seconds before applying moisturiser. Bedtime is a good time to do this, as morning use will dictate that you must follow your moisturiser with a sunblock to prevent potential damage.

SERUM

Serum's job is to treat any existing skin conditions or complaints. It's very fine in texture and usually laden with anti-ageing ingredients. There are thousands on the market, so read the packaging carefully to ensure a product is designed for your specific concerns – such as dehydration, age spots and uneven pigmentation, wrinkles, oiliness, and so on.

There are some excellent multi-purpose serums by Estée Lauder, Clinique, Olay, Nivea, L'Oréal Paris, Vichy and Clarins. You may like to use a different one at night to the morning.

After either cleansing or exfoliating, massage a couple of drops into the face, including around the eye area. You can be firm here. Wait a few seconds before applying any other creams or oils.

MOISTURISERS – DAY AND NIGHT

Moisturisers can be either creams or oils and are designed to comfort and protect your skin, and prepare it for make-up. A good one will make skin look and feel instantly better than before. Do not be tempted to skip this step if you have oily skin – every type benefits from moisture and the least helpful thing you can do for your skin is deliberately starve it (this is actually counterproductive as oily skin will often just pump out more oil to lubricate itself). I believe moisturiser is an essential step, but not that the moisturiser itself needs to be fancy.

A cream needs to lubricate your skin (not cause it to break out), leave it comfortable and keep it protected. It's not capable of a great deal more so beware of marketing hype.

When choosing a moisturiser, check first that it is designed for your particular skin type. There are oils, lotions and creams for every condition. I like creams and lotions by Neutrogena, Simple, Estée Lauder, Clarins, REN, Revive, Olay, Darphin, Carita, Murad, Sisley and many more. The more important thing is that you use it. I would also check the packaging to ensure a moisturiser contains no mineral oil, which can aggravate the spot-prone. I don't personally have a problem with mineral oil, other than that it's cheap and there are nicer alternatives which I would expect brands who are pocketing your cash to use more widely.

My favourite oils are by Clarins, Decléor, Neal's Yard, Trilogy, Pai, Sunday Riley, Balance Me and those available from health-food stores.

After serum, massage in moisturiser firmly but gently. It's perfectly fine to include your eye area and skip eye cream, as long as your eyes aren't irritated by this.

NAPPY RASH CREAM

There are times when skin flares up, and while it's important to examine what caused it (allergies, hormones, poor diet, snogging a stubbly man), it's also necessary to clear it up. Nappy rash cream serves no long-term purpose but does its specific job very swiftly and effectively. It's generally very white and very unctuous, though, so apply at night or when slobbing around one's own nest away from public gaze.

My favourite ointment is by Kiehl's but to be perfectly honest, most nappy creams will do the job reasonably well.

Apply generously over spots and redness after your nighttime serum.

SUNBLOCK

You know you're supposed to use it, so please do so. Sunblock is a must and probably the most powerful tool we have in the war against skin damage and premature ageing. There are two types of sunblock: physical and chemical. Physical is ideal for kids and sensitive-skinned adults, but can feel greasy, look chalky and provide a very poor base for make-up. If you can tolerate either chemical or a chemical/physical mix, I'd recommend it. (For more on sunblocks, see Anti-ageing.)

I like facial sunblocks from Prevage, Clinique, Ultrasun, Shu Uemura, Zelens, La Roche Posay, Intraceuticals, Simple, Estée Lauder and Shiseido, but any broad-spectrum sunblock (that's one that protects against both UVA and UVB) with an SPF of 30+ will work (the difference between an SPF30 and SPF50 is tiny).

In summer months, apply after cleansing and before make-up. In autumn and winter, you can either use a day cream containing sun SPF15 or above, or use a foundation or tinted moisturiser with added sun protection.

LIP BALM

I have lip balms everywhere – in every bag and coat, in every room, in the ashtray and glove compartment of my car. It's always good to have one on standby for when lips feel dry, breath feels stale, lipstick looks uneven, or I just need a little pick-me-up.

I am an equal opportunities balm addict. I use super-cheap, mega-spendy and everything in between. I am also very fickle, falling in love with one, then a week later dumping it for another. Those I return to quite frequently include Maybelline, Clinique, Carmex, Perfumeria Gal, Crème de La Mer, Aerin, Kiehl's, MAC, Korres and Lanolips.

Apply with your ring finger or straight from a tube around twice a day or whenever lips feel dry.

Tinted moisturiser

Tinted moisturisers make everyone look better. They are, in my opinion, infinitely superior to BB (blemish balm) creams because they give a lovely healthy glow to the skin. (See Foundation for more information on tinted moisturisers.)

My favourite tinted moisturisers are by Origins, Laura Mercier, Chantecaille, Nivea, Becca and Nars.

After serum, dot tinted moisturiser on the nose, cheeks, chin and forehead and blend into skin. If your skin is particularly dry, you will need to moisturise first with a day cream (I do).

Concealer

I don't care who you are, you absolutely need a concealer, and when you try it, you'll never turn back. Concealer evens out dark patches, covers spots, disguises under-eye circles and generally makes you look about a hundred times better. It needs to match your skin tone or, failing that, be a fraction lighter, and be creamy and opaque to do its job properly. It should contain light-reflecting particles to counteract dark circles, but is not to be confused with those highlighting pens, though everyone seems to make this mistake.

The best multi-purpose concealers are by Nars, MAC, Laura Mercier, Amazing Cosmetics, Clarins and Bobbi Brown. All but Clarins make them for both light and dark skins.

Dot concealer under your eyes, over spots and on any areas of redness (around the nose is a common hotspot). Using your ring finger, gently pat in the concealer, feathering it outwards, then set with powder. To cover a particularly evil spot, follow my instruction in the Bridal chapter.

Powder

Powder is so underrated; I think because women are commonly told that it is ageing, when it really isn't. What powder does, uniquely, is lock make-up down, stopping it from taking a walk during the day. It also banishes shine, which, ironically, I find quite ageing. Gleam and dewiness are young and bright, yes, but shine? No. No one wants to look as though they are in the throes of a hot flash or an anxiety attack. Powder also gives a sort of pulled-together polish to a finished face and is the fastest way to revive make-up during the day. It needs to match your skin tone exactly. There are translucent powders designed to suit everyone, but I'm decidedly unkeen. I use loose powder at home, pressed for touch-ups, but if we're talking essentials, go for a pressed powder compact and you'll always be prepared.

The best powders are by Bobbi Brown, Chantecaille, Bourjois, Urban Decay, Charlotte Tilbury, Chanel, T. LeClerc, Max Factor and MAC.

After any other base – primer, foundation, tinted moisturiser or concealer – pat on powder with a velour puff (the one in the compact is fine), then sweep over a fat brush to remove any excess.

A MATTE IVORY AND A SLIGHTLY SHIMMERY BROWN EYESHADOW

Everyone looks good in brown eyeshadow, which is handy, as it's the easiest to put on. Brown goes with everything and gives warmth and depth to all skin tones. It also doubles as a suits-everyone eyeliner. Ivory is a very useful tone for all colourings and gives a smooth, brightening base onto which you can pop any other colour.

Brand is not terribly important here. I personally rate Bourjois, Bobbi Brown, MAC, Burberry Beauty, Dior, Chanel, Tom Ford, Charlotte Tilbury, Nars, Clarins and Sleek, but the main thing is to get the colour and finish right. Your ivory needs to be sparkle free so that anything can be blended over the top. Your brown needs to be dark and with a slight shimmer for easy blending and softness.

Apply the ivory with a large eyeshadow brush, from lash line to brow, before using any other shadow. To add brown, take a crease brush (the shape of a fat cotton bud or Q-tip and made from natural bristles) and with a windscreen wipers action, sweep back and forth into your eyelid crease, then move downwards, washing the colour over the lid. To use as a liner, take a small liner brush and trace the brown shadow around your lash line, top and bottom.

BLACK MASCARA

Or brown if you prefer, though I cannot quite see the point. In any case, mascara makes a huge difference on everyone. If you are a smudger (I am – it comes from having to wear very rich moisturiser under my eyes. Fiddlers and weepers will also suffer), then you'll need a tubing mascara, made from polymers that coat each lash in a sort of plastic tube. They are less dramatic than traditional mascaras, but they simply don't budge until you wash them off with warm water. If smudging is not an issue, the world's your oyster and you can buy whichever mascara appeals.

The best tubing mascaras are by Estée Lauder, Clinique, Sensai, Kevyn Aucoin, Eyeko and L'Oréal Paris.

The best of the traditional mascaras are by Lancôme, L'Oréal Paris, YSL, Maybelline, Dior, MAC and Charlotte Tilbury.

In either case, you need to first stroke the wand downwards over the top of your lashes, then upwards on the underside, using a zig-zagging motion to separate them. Use what's left on the wand for your lower lashes, using the same motion. Dip the wand back in for your second eye. Wait a few moments then repeat for a second coat.

PINK OR APRICOT BLUSHER

Either shade is fine. I switch back and forth to match to the undertones of my lipstick, but those with rosy cheeks may prefer to stick to apricot. The darker your skin, the darker you may go. Formulation – whether creme or powder – is also a matter of preference. The former gives a soft, natural flush while the latter looks more polished and has greater longevity. What is more important is that there is some colour there. Blusher is an absolute non-negotiable for me. It adds a youthful glow to all skin tones (blusher is certainly not only for the pale) and makes you look perkier and healthier.

Brand is your call. I personally like creme blushers by Liz Earle, Tarte, Aerin, Clarins, Bourjois, MAC, Max Factor and Bobbi Brown. For powders I visit Nars, Charlotte Tilbury, Bourjois, Bobbi Brown,

Smashbox, Chanel and Tom Ford.

For creme blush, apply three dots of colour to the fat part of your cheeks, then blend in a circle with your middle finger. Finish by using a clean fingertip to blend the outer side of the circle into a tear-drop shape.

For powder blush, take a fat blusher brush with a rounded edge (never use the one in the compact – it will be rubbish) and stroke it over the powder blush pan, on both brush sides and the tip, coating the bristles evenly. Stroke the brush onto a clean tissue or your hand to remove excess. Smile, and stroke the brush along the fat parts of your cheeks, blending outwards. Do not go too far and 'take off' up to your ears or you will look stripy and weird.

A NUDE LIPSTICK

When I say nude, I never mean the wholly prejudicial industry standard of generic beige. I mean any colour that could conceivably be the colour of natural lips (or complexion, in the case of eyeshadows and blusher), from rosy pink to mauve to chocolate brown. A nude lipstick goes with any eyeshadow, outfit or occasion and is neither under nor overdressed. If you have very thin lips or just really, really can't deal with lipstick then a tinted balm or gloss is fine. Though even then, I would still say we'll all be dead soon – just put on some lipstick while you still can. You will look lovely.

I wear lipsticks by anyone and everyone. Go for any brand you like, but do choose a satiny finish as your everyday lipstick. Matte looks cool but needs to be applied perfectly and can be more of a statement than one necessarily feels like making on a daily basis. Frosty is reliably horrible, it makes lips look flaky and any woman appear as though she has no knowledge of fashion post-1985.

Optional extras

These items aren't essential but are good to have, depending on your beauty concerns.

A face mask

It's nice to give your skin a midweek boost or treatment. I enjoy using masks for this. I like how my skin feels afterwards, but because of a solid everyday skincare routine, I don't feel bereft if I skip it here and there. Choose a mask that addresses your particular skincare concern. I favour those containing large doses of hyaluronic acid that will hydrate my skin and plump it back up, but you could instead opt for a spot treatment mask or an intense exfoliant.

I love masks by Sisley, Origins, Astalift, SKII, Sarah Chapman, REN, Aveda, Estée Lauder, Zelens, Skyn Iceland and Soap and Glory to name but a few.

Application guidelines vary wildly from mask to mask, so follow the instructions on the packaging. My only general guideline is to always start with clean skin and if the mask is to be removed (rather than left to absorb), this is best done with a hot cloth.

Lip pencil

Lip pencils stop lipstick bleed and define your lip line, which gets fuzzier over time. They also give a neater finish to any lip colour. It's essential that your liner matches either your lipstick or your naked lips. If you can't match, choose a clear one (Body Shop, Estée Lauder, MAC and Cargo make these). Don't be tempted to contrast, ever. MAC, Estée Lauder, Rimmel and Bobbi Brown make the best coloured lip pencils.

Brow powder or crayon

If your brows are sparse or paler than you'd like, you may want to fill them in with brow colour. I never bother if I'm having a casual day, but I always fill in brows if I'm wearing foundation and eyeshadow. Do not use a pencil to do this, though – they're too harsh. I like those by Suqqu, Anastasia, Tom Ford, Lancôme, Sleek and Bourjois.

Dark brown eyeliner pencil

If you can't be bothered with the hassle of carrying a liner brush and powder, get a chocolate-brown eyeliner pencil. The colour suits everyone, goes with every look and is smart, yet soft. It will define your eyes and make them appear more open and white. Line around the upper and lower lashlines, smudging the lower with your little finger before applying mascara. Among my favourites are those by Clinique, Elizabeth Arden, Givenchy, Charlotte Tilbury and Bourjois.

Bronzer

Do not fear bronzer. The correct one is your friend. When the colour is just a couple of shades darker than your own, without being orange or muddy brown, then you're halfway there. Its job is to add a healthy looking glow to any skin tone (black skins benefit just as much from bronzer as white), contour and depth of field to the complexion. I personally am never without it, though I appreciate it is, to some, one step too many in the morning.

On white skins I like bronzers by Aerin, Bourjois, Burberry, Sisley, Guerlain and Bobbi Brown. For brown and black skins I like MAC, Nars, Guerlain, YSL, L'Oréal Paris and Rimmel.

Apply bronzer in figure '3's after the base but before blush. By that I mean start at your temples, moving downwards, coming into your cheeks as though you are drawing a figure '3', then out again to your jawline. Do the same in mirror image on the other side. Then apply blusher. It looks gorgeous.

Things you don't need

I believe these products to be either a nonsense or an unnecessary extravagance. Spend your money where you'll see the benefit.

Anti-cellulite creams, gels, serums – yada, yada ...

I personally believe these to be the snake oils of the beauty industry and feel they are always best left alone. They are expensive, boring to apply and, most significantly, I cannot see how they can possibly work, however many research studies I'm shown. Invest in a good body scrub and a wash-off tan. Both will minimise the look of cellulite better than anything else I've seen. No product can rid you of cellulite.

Bust gels

Bust-growth gels make me crosser than almost anything. They are, I believe, a nonsense. No topical product can penetrate the skin to create fat cells (breasts are made of fatty tissue). The very idea makes no sense whatsoever. Buy some removable silicone chicken fillets, try a push-up bra or learn to love your tits. I strongly believe that no cream will ever make the slightest difference.

Anything claiming to act as a 'detox'

What balls. I would cheerfully ban this silly word if I could. Beauty products can reduce bacteria, affect pH balance, soothe, calm, cleanse – lots of good things – but they cannot 'detoxify' beyond the superficial. The structure of your skin will not be altered by products, and nor will the tissue beneath it. This is cod science invented to shift product and can safely be ignored.

EYE CREAM

My relationship with eye cream is not clear-cut, so let me explain. You need a form of moisturiser around your eye area and eye cream is marvellous at doing this without irritation. However, it is still, when all is said and done, an anti-ageing moisturiser sold in a tiny pot and not the magic product the beauty industry implies it to be. So if you suffer no adverse reactions from using your regular anti-ageing day cream around your eyes, and no puffiness occurs, then you are perfectly fine to use it all over and not bother with an eye cream. However, if you do find your day cream too rich for your eyes, then by all means buy a separate cream for the area. I like eye creams by Estée Lauder, Zelens, Olay, L'Oréal Paris and Clinique.

NECK CREAMS

For much the same reasons as above, I don't believe anyone really needs a neck cream. A firming moisturiser will do just as well, although, frankly, no cream will dramatically tighten a sagging neck. The best way to prevent this happening in the first place is to include your neck in your daily routine (not getting dressed until you've put on your skincare helps avoid omission), to wear good broad-spectrum sun protection when your neck and chest is uncovered and to not smoke. If damage has already occurred (or even if it hasn't) you can try exercising the underlying muscles to create better scaffolding for the skin above them. (See Anti-ageing for more on this.) If the situation is drastic, you have three choices: plastic surgery, self-acceptance or lovely cashmere polo-neck jumpers. The third seems most appealing.

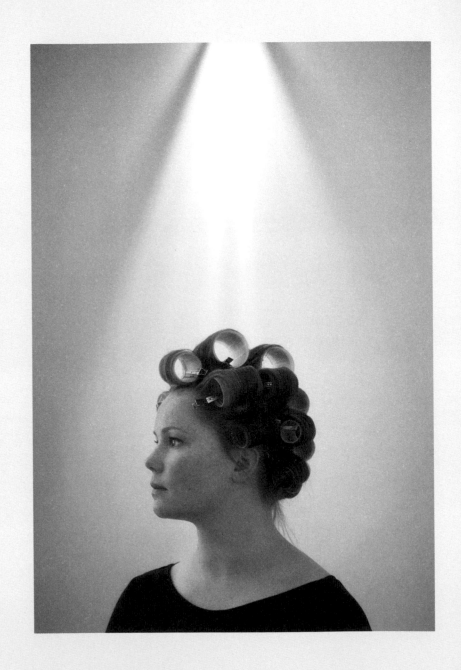

SALON ETIQUETTE

'I think that the most important thing a women can have next to talent, of course, is her hairdresser.'
Joan Crawford

I have always loved going to the hair or beauty salon. Chiefly because I spent my first seven or so years being taken along with my brothers for identical bowl cuts from bemused old men in the local barbershop. Between the truly dire cuts, my father would sweetly stand me on a kitchen chair and attempt to put my hair in bunches, snapping several elastics (he had to buy them by the two-dozen, still on their display card from the chemist) and filling the room with profanity. When we eventually moved in with my mother and she took me to her salon, I loved it instantly and deeply.

I've never outgrown it and still see salons as lovely, transformative havens from everyday annoyance. People playing with my hair while I sip on tea or champagne and flick through magazines, or a nice woman treating my face to a deep cleanse and massage while I drift off to sleep to the sound of whalesong – how could anyone not want an appointment? But I'm no longer surprised when I hear people say they dread a salon visit. Invariably, I find that women and men see salon appointments as a tip-toe across a minefield of salon etiquette that one is supposed to implicitly understand without having ever been told. I've visited more hair and beauty salons than tube stations and, admittedly, with occasionally dire results (Lady Di flicks on a permed mullet being one of the greater traumas). I understand the common trepidation and I know the rules.

Allow me to demystify the experience with the basic code of salon conduct. It will help you to enjoy a blissful salon experience that allows you to get exactly the look you want.

KEY SALON ETIQUETTE

Dilemma

You want to read your book, they want to chat.

Solution

Guess what? They almost certainly don't want to chat and would much sooner be getting on with things – they're just trying to be friendly, as is expected. Exchange niceties, then politely say you'd like to do some reading while you have the rare chance of a break, or that you have work to do on your laptop. They honestly won't mind. If you're having a facial, massage or any other relaxing beauty treatment, a running commentary is completely not on. Say politely and firmly that you've been looking forward to some quiet relaxation and you're sorry to not be feeling chatty on this occasion. If the therapist persists, give feedback to the manager and don't tip – a chatty massage is the absolute pits.

Dilemma

The therapist you're offered is more senior than you can afford. Are senior staff that much better that you should suck up the cost?

Solution

A stylist or therapist's rank is an indicator of experience. Very generally speaking, the higher the rank, the greater the number of clients they've treated and the techniques they've studied. That said, a junior stylist may absolutely do an equal, or even better job than someone more senior. If money is tight, save your high-flyer money for dramatic restyles or major treatments only. For trims, nail-paint jobs and blow dries in between, see someone cheaper. If the more junior therapist does a consistently great job, move over to him/her for everything.

Dilemma

You feel uncomfortable.

Solution

Life is too short and money too precious to waste either in a salon you don't like or with people you don't want to deal with. I have walked out of umpteen salons (some of them very expensive) in my lifetime, sometimes with wet hair or while hastily doing up my jeans. If a salon seems grubby, leave. If the staff are rude, leave. If you feel like you don't matter, leave (if the lighting makes you look awful, I'm afraid you will have to learn to accept that all salon lighting is unfathomably ghastly, and stay). There are brilliant salons who need your business, so get the hell out of there and find one – a personal recommendation from someone with great hair / skin / nails (as appropriate) is always best.

Dilemma
You're a pounder, they're a stroker.
Solution
There is nothing worse than a mimsy massage or facial, if like me, you've gone purely to enjoy a good hammering. I want to feel body or face muscles being worked, gross stuff being extracted from my skin. Being stroked by a therapist (one facialist even spent 45 minutes with her hands floating above my face to cleanse my aura) makes me so unrelaxed that I leave feeling murderous. But unless you tell the therapist what you're after, how can they know? Tell them cheerfully upon arrival that you like a firm or light pressure, that your pain threshold is high or low, and let them know at any point in the treatment if they've gone too far in either direction. It's also useful to express your preferences when booking the initial appointment. Most salons will have a therapist with a firmer or softer touch than others and will be happy to match you accordingly.

Dilemma
You want to dump your hairdresser or therapist.
Solution
There comes a time when a beauty professional / client relationship, however happy once, becomes stale. Hairstyles become samey and tired, massage gets half-arsed. Sometimes, the therapist is promoted through the ranks and becomes unaffordable. It's time to move on to pastures new. This can be mortifying if you move to a different

practitioner in the same salon because no one wants to stride past the rejected party, new stylist in tow. I would move salons, if possible, but if you are really mustard-keen on someone at the same place, then brave it out. Make a point of saying hello to your former professional, ask how they are – for God's sake, don't pretend you can't see them. When they ask who you're with today, tell them, smile and say that you felt like a change for a bit. Never, ever criticise the former stylist or therapist to the new one. It's naff.

Dilemma
You never know which way the gown goes on.
Solution
Like a coat. You are confusing the salon with the operating theatre. No one has used back-tying gowns since 1982.

Dilemma
Is taking in photographs rude?
Solution
Hell, no. Visual reference materials are almost always preferred by hairdressers and make-up artists. They save so much time otherwise spent attempting to explain a look verbally, and leave little room for misunderstanding. They are essential and most stylists are secretly frustrated when a client doesn't bring visual references. Search for photographs on the internet and print them out, tear pictures from magazines, bring in snaps of yourself wearing a look you'd like to revisit.

Dilemma
Should you pay for the head massage and do you even have to have it?
Solution
No, on both counts. Your hair washer may well hope to be tipped for a head massage but you are not obliged to (though I would, massage or none – see 'Tipping' box). You certainly needn't accept a massage you don't want. The washer should always ask and a simple 'yes please' or 'no thank you' is quite enough. Don't try to explain yourself.

Dilemma

Can you use your phone during a treatment?

Solution

I personally think it's rude to gab away to a third party while someone is attempting to concentrate on your nails, feet, hair or mons pubis. I mean, really, is it that important you chat to others while a stranger sees to your labia? By all means let the therapist know you need to take an important call, but then tell the caller you're in the salon and it's inconvenient. It's the correct thing to do.

Dilemma

Is it okay to accept Champagne or wine?

Solution

If it's free, it's offered to you and you fancy it, say thank you and enjoy it. If it were gauche to accept, it would be gauche of them to offer. I sometimes find, though, that alcohol makes for a dizzying and ultimately less relaxing facial or massage, and that a glass of wine + tuggy blow dry = headache, but each to her own. I certainly find a glass of something fizzy towards the end of the day raises my spirits and propels me forward to a night out in a giddier frame of mind.

Dilemma

Your hairdresser or therapist has moved salons.

Solution

When a therapist moves to another salon, the professional protocol is that they neither announce they're leaving, nor say where they're going. This is extremely frustrating when you go to book your next appointment and the receptionist gets all tight-lipped about where the hell your favourite is now working. This is why I always, always find out the full name of hairstylists and beauty therapists I love. That way, you can search Facebook and Instagram and get in touch direct. As long as you're approaching them and not vice versa, no one is out of line.

Dilemma
You hate your hair.
Solution
Be extremely clear about what you want from the start and always take photographs with you, printed out from the internet or torn from magazines (see above). This not only gives you a better chance of getting the hair you want, but also gives you a leg to stand on if you don't. If the stylist took off three inches when you agreed on one, say so. If your colour is brassy when you agreed on golden, say it will need to be fixed. If they give you that weird Lulu / Judy Finnegan haircut so many stylists consider to be the default for women over 40, ask them to blunt off the layers. The more you can get nailed down in consultation the better.

Dilemma
No, seriously, you really, really hate your hair.
Solution
If your stylist or colourist has either ignored your wishes or caused unnecessary damage to your hair or skin, and fails to fix the problem, then it's time to get serious. Send them a clear, unemotional letter letting them know you are taking them to small claims court (see www. adviceguide.org.uk for advice on how to do this), giving the salon 14 days to respond and offer a resolution. Don't be insulting or personal. If you hear nothing in response, follow through on your promise and let the court handle it.

Tipping

Americans obviously have this pretty nailed, but we Europeans struggle with the gratuities minefield. This is how it works: if you are happy with your hair/facial/massage/wax and the service you received, then a tip is nice. I generally tip 10–15 per cent of the total. If it's a hairdressing tip then I immediately ringfence £5 from the tip and give it to whoever washed my hair (they suffer sore, irritated hands, wash towels, sweep floors, massage heads and basically work like dogs for terrible money). I give the remainder to the therapist or stylist. If there is also a colourist, I split the remainder clean in half between them. I tip everyone via the receptionist and tell her/him how much is for whom. It takes seconds. The receptionist will then envelope and mark up the tips and distribute them (I discourage personal tipping since walking across to the basins waving a fiver is a bit gauche). Using percentages means you never have to think about the inherent 'value' in a stylist's status and whether to factor that in – everyone, from junior stylist to creative director gets the same percentage. It's much simpler. The only exception to this rule is if your stylist or therapist is the salon owner, in which case I would never tip unless they are running a tiny enterprise.

And stripping

People panic over which items of clothing to remove in salons. A good therapist will be clear and explicit, but here's a cheat sheet for when they aren't.

Classic bikini wax
Tights and trousers off. Knickers on (unless they give
you paper underwear to change into).

....

Hollywood or Brazilian bikini wax
Tights, trousers and knickers off (unless you're given paper knickers),
a courtesy cleanse with a baby wipe before treatment.

Body massage
All clothing, jewellery and bra off. Knickers on.

....

Spray or self-tan
All clothing, jewellery and bra off. Paper knickers on –
a good salon will not expect you to ruin your own.

....

Reflexology
Tights, socks, jeans off. Underwear on.

....

Facial
Top and jewellery off, bra on (though the therapist will probably
lower the straps during the treatment).

....

Leg waxing
All clothing below the waist removed, underwear on.

....

Manicure
Sleeves rolled up. Get your payment method out in advance.

....

Pedicure
Socks removed, trousers rolled up. Take flip-flops.

....

Head massage
No changing required at hair salon or public space. For salon massage
with oils, remove jewellery and clothing from the waist up, but leave bra on.

....

Saunas and steam rooms
Check specific club policy. Many encourage swimming
briefs, many allow nudity.

....

Sunbeds
Stop using them.

WHEN THE SALON KNOWS BEST

Yes, it's your money but you are paying for expertise. It's often worth shutting up and listening. Here are some examples of when the hairdresser's word is law.

'We need to skin test before making any colour appointment'
Allergies to hair dye can cause grave harm to clients and sometimes even kill. Hair salons don't want this to happen and nor should you. Don't argue if your colourist demands a skin test in advance of any colour appointments – it's a good sign of a responsible salon and will give you a better indication of how you'll respond to the dye (not being allergic last year is neither here nor there. Hair dye allergies can develop after many years of safe dyeing).

'It won't look exactly like it does in the picture because...'
Hairstyles are not a one-suits-all business. Everything needs to be adapted and expectations must be managed. Clearly, no one with thick, curly hair is going to be able to pull off a Louise Brooks bob without a little tinkering, and nor is someone with my fine, flat hair likely to replicate a photo of Beyoncé. Save yourself the disappointment later by listening to your stylist now. They know what your hair is capable of.

'Your hair needs a break from permanent colour'
Hairdressers spend their lives looking at hair. They know the difference between healthy locks and those on the verge of snapping in two or falling clean out. When a colourist calls time on chemical processing, be thankful they warned you and take the break.

'Uncross your legs'
A stylist who asks you to sit up straight with uncrossed legs is looking out for you – an unbalanced frame can very easily result in a wonky haircut.

'That won't suit your face shape'
If you spend every day staring at faces in mirrors, watching them transform from round to heart-shaped thanks to a few jaw-grazing layers, you develop a pretty good sense of which styles work on whom. If your stylist says a super-short blunt fringe will make your face look fat, they are probably right. Let them cut in a sweepier version instead.

THINGS YOU NEVER NEED TO ACCEPT

You are the customer and some of your expectations are, frankly, non-negotiable. Adopt a zero-tolerance policy on these.

'Conditioner costs extra'
It is not wartime. Hair conditioner is not some rare, exotic elixir. Charging for conditioner is the beauty equivalent of serving orange juice as a starter.

'I'll just get you gowned and washed then Kate will be over to look at your hair'
I don't trust any stylist who decides what to do with my hair while I'm sitting, soaking wet and covered in a huge gown. A good hairdresser looks at how you dress, how your hair is styled and falls naturally, how you carry yourself. This is your hair – it needs to look good on you, not against the salon wallpaper.

Tea and coffee charges
No. If you want something special, like champagne, a panini or a slab of cake, then a charge is reasonable. But basic refreshments of tea, coffee and mineral water while sitting in the chair should always, always be free and unlimited.

'We only go with the natural hair texture'
I'm alarmed when I (increasingly often) hear this in European hair salons (you'd never hear it in Afro-Caribbean salons). Frankly, if you won't curl straight hair or blow-dry curly hair straight then you should really consider a change of career. For me, the job of a hair salon is to perform things I am not skilled enough to do at home. That means, amongst other things, giving my poker-straight hair a bit of shape. If I wanted to look entirely natural, I'd save my £70 and stay home.

'We don't do consultations'
Oh really? So you just give every client an identical cut then? A consultation needn't last longer than a few minutes but should always be available and free. This is where you and your stylist discuss the cut you want, look at photographs, consider any adaptations, whether the style will be achievable at home and so on. A consultation is essential when considering a restyle (if you always see the same stylist and are just having a trim, then you can skip it).

Tutting, sniggering and eye rolling
I'm amazed at how often I hear friends complaining of this. Each to her own, but I'm not okay with salon staff criticising other clients and co-workers on the shop floor. Why? Because it makes me paranoid that I'm next. Gossip should be kept clean, fun and strictly celebrity-based.

'MODELLING': WHAT TO EXPECT

Many salons will hang signs saying 'Models Wanted'. This is not an opportunity for stardom, but the possibility of a free or extremely cheap haircut or beauty treatment. Models are used for training young hairstylists (sometimes already qualified ones), who will already have done a fair bit of cutting practice on wigs and dummies. Beauty therapist trainees have usually performed treatments on friends and relatives. If you agree to model, check your trainee will be supervised by a qualified practitioner and that any techniques – hair colouring or bikini waxing, for example – aren't entirely new to them. Expect to pay either around 20–50 per cent of the normal price, or nothing at all. Avoid modelling if you want a total hair restyle – subtle changes are less risky. Things like hair trims, manicures, pedicures, facials and massage are safest. Local college courses in hair and beauty often use models too, so look them up.

Warning
In any modelling situation, expect to be there for at least twice as long as in a conventional salon setting. Trainees are understandably slower when taking instruction and being assessed, so don't be the intolerant person who makes a fuss. Get a time estimate in advance and take a good book.

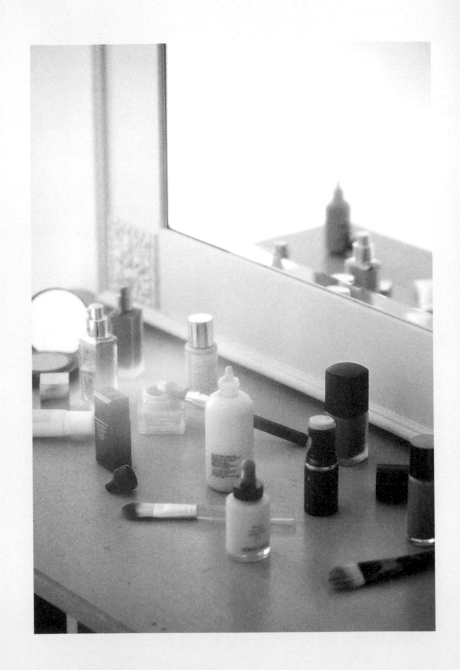

FOUNDATION

'The best thing is to look natural,
but it takes make-up to look natural.'
Calvin Klein

Time and time again, mascara is found to be most women's most indispensable product, but I disagree. Good-looking skin is everything in beauty, not least because it occupies the largest expanse of facial real estate. A good base really does make a huge difference to your overall appearance and I believe every woman should own one – even if they wear it only on special occasions. Yet foundation, the most transformative of make-up products, is the one most women get wrong, either thanks to appalling department-store lighting or pushy sales people insistent on 'warming you up' (if you hear this, run). There's also quite often some degree of mental scarring thanks to the horrific, trowelled-on orange pastes of yore, still putting women off years later.

I spent my eleventh and twelfth years attending school in a Mary Quant foundation the colour of window putty, spread all over my face with a rancid wedge sponge, obscuring my then-completely-clear complexion (I also covered my lips to the point where they practically disappeared from my face – strong look). As the day wore on, it crawled onto my many dry patches and sort of died there. I see photographs now and could slap myself in the face (the foundation would have covered the bruising and then some). I'm amazed to find this look endures today on grown women.

It makes me sad when I see a teenager with plump, even, peachy skin swathed in thick foundation, but to be entirely honest, this is the only time I discourage base. The rest of us will benefit enormously from a great foundation. A great base is your best friend. It unifies uneven colour tone, melding age spots and sun damage into one consistent colour. This makes skin look younger and vibrant. The aim is always to make the skin look the best it possibly can, without ever seeming unnatural. A great foundation's job is to perfect the skin, making you appear clearer, brighter, more youthful and never, ever as though dipped in Ronseal. It should look like skin, not make-up. Basically, foundation should be a wholly convincing con trick.

So why does foundation get such a bad rap? I meet women who are terrified of wearing it, who associate foundation with dull, matte, cakey complexions in implausible shades of tan beige (I have known possibly five women in my lifetime with the classic 'medium' skin tone that brands seem to believe is so widespread). Women have come home, time and time again, having spent the cost of a decent babysitter on an unwearable foundation that suits no one but an earthenware tagine. And how women of colour manage to leave the department stores without attacking a make-up counter with their handbag is beyond me, so under-served or plainly ignored are they by very many brands (especially those from Japan, whose ranges rarely go darker than pale olive, shamefully).

Even women who win the foundation lottery and come home with something in the right colour seem to fall at the second hurdle – application. The finish is textured like satsuma peel, not smooth like an egg. It sits in wrinkles, instead of blurring them. It's thick-looking, patchy, mask-like, or wanders off the face within an hour of putting it on. It looks fine on the face, bloody awful against the neck. It causes me to despair at the lost opportunity to look better than you've looked in years. Trust me, foundation can be more fabulous than anything, with a little know-how.

How to choose a foundation

Before we tread the colour minefield, there's the more pressing matter of formulation. There is no point choosing a foundation without carefully considering what you need it to do for you. In order to do that, you must first establish your skin type (see What's Your Skin Type?), then decide which formula is right for your needs and grooming levels.

BB (BLEMISH BALM) CREAM

Suitable for
Young, oily and combination skins. Fans of low-maintenance beauty and those with little time for grooming.

Not suitable for
Dry, dehydrated or mature skins.

I am not a fan, but I seem to be the only one, so I should explain. The idea behind BBs is that they perform the task of a sunblock, moisturiser, sheer foundation and spot treatment, all in one cream. For many – especially the young or those pushed for time in the mornings – this is quite an attractive proposition. In reality, I think while decent at sun protection, they deliver quite badly on the moisturiser and foundation side of the bargain. They offer nowhere near enough moisture or hydration to dry and dehydrated skins, such as mine. Wearing them alone leaves dry skin tight and flaky, in my experience. They also, at time of writing, mostly deliver a very flat, matte, almost clay-like finish to the skin, making them extremely unflattering on older skins without enough natural glow to overpower it. Finally, so, so few cater for non-Caucasian skin, which I resent. They either don't match any black or Asian skins, or when they do, have such a chalky finish that they make any dark tone appear ashy. BB creams will get better, I'm sure, but in 2014, I'm seeing few encouraging signs (but a whole generation of devotees – I do realise I'm outnumbered here).

If there were a gun to my head, I'd tell you to buy BBs by Bobbi Brown and Estée Lauder.

CC (COLOUR CORRECTING) CREAMS
Suitable for
Most skin types and ages.
Not suitable for
Very dry or very dehydrated skins.

A similar idea to BB creams. A multi-function product that protects against the sun, moisturises and acts as a sheer foundation. The CC stands for colour correcting – the point being to blend in sunspots, melasma and other pigmentation problems, though so far I've only found a couple that do this well (foundations are better at this). Overall, I've found them to be a little more moisturising than BB creams, making them more comfortable on dry and dehydrated skins, though still not enough for those on the far end of either scale. They can work very well at camouflaging uneven tone and have a slightly sheerer finish than BBs. I will wear one of these occasionally, out of curiosity, whereas I wouldn't put a BB on my face unless it were the last product in my bathroom.

The best CCs, for me, are by Clinique, Darphin, Origins, Smashbox and Bobbi Brown (all owned by Estée Lauder, which I feel is no coincidence).

TINTED MOISTURISER

Suitable for
Everyone (use oil-free on oily skins for staying power), summertime, casual days.
Not suitable for
Severely blemished or unevenly toned skin.

What, in my view, BB creams should be. A sheer, glowing, healthy-looking base for a fresh and natural look. TMs are for days when you don't want to feel made up but you do want to look better. Good ones offer some coverage and contain sun protection and light reflectors for faux glow. Don't take the name on trust, though. If you have dry skin, tinted moisturisers can very rarely replace a regular moisturiser and are better applied at the foundation stage. Most can only be worn solo if you have enough natural oil in your skin to remain comfortable (if you're very oily, choose an oil-free formula for staying power). If dry, smooth on day cream first then wait a few moments before following with a tinted moisturiser and concealer, if required. Laura Mercier makes the best, but I also rate Origins, Chantecaille, Nivea and Becca's versions.

SHEER FOUNDATION

Suitable for
Clear skins, anyone who wants a very natural look, women with freckles.
Not suitable for
Severely blemished skin.

Usually liquid in texture, a sheer foundation is basically like holding a 5-denier stocking over your face. Coverage is very light and natural-looking, helping to unify skin tone but not covering any redness or acne. Best applied with either fingertips or a foundation brush (sheer foundations are usually so thin in texture that sponges just drink them up, wasting loads of product), they can usually be layered for denser coverage. To do this, apply, then wait a few moments before applying more where needed. Armani, Revlon, Becca and Dior make fantastic sheer bases for all ethnicities.

LIQUID FOUNDATION

Suitable for
Everyone (oily skins should opt for an oil-free liquid formula for better staying power).

The default foundation type, and one with medium coverage – that is, it will blend out any unevenness and light blemishes, but still look natural in the right colour. Liquid is extremely versatile and there is one for every skin type. If you're dry, look for a moisturising formula (Bobbi Brown's is superb), if dull, go for one with light reflectors (Stila, Charlotte Tilbury and YSL are brilliant for this). Armani, Bobbi Brown and MAC are unusually good in terms of catering for a wide range of skin tones. All liquids can be applied with a brush, fingers or sponge (I favour a brush). If you are buying your first foundation, I say buy a liquid.

MINERAL FOUNDATION POWDER

Suitable for
Sensitive skins, those with rosacea, acne or women who have neither the time nor the inclination to cleanse thoroughly before bed.
Not suitable for
Dull skins.

Mineral foundations have become massively popular in the past decade. Made of crushed-up natural minerals and other cosmetic ingredients, they're applied with a large brush and buffed into moisturised skin. They fill a previously neglected gap in the market, servicing women whose skin is extremely sensitive to make-up, and can give natural, buildable coverage. My only reservation is that they can look quite 'flat' and dull on the skin. Dull, sallow skin types are best with a different formulation, if possible. My favourites are by Neal's Yard, Laura Mercier, Jane Iredale and Bare Minerals.

CREAM FOUNDATION

Suitable for
Dry, normal, combination or heavily blemished skins.
Not suitable for
Oily and young skins.

I love cream foundation. It's brilliant for dressy evenings out when you might want your skin to look flawless and is extremely comfortable on dry or mature skins. Applied properly (sparingly), it gives a moist, flattering glow but medium to full coverage, covering up discolouration and light blemishes. My favourites are by Suqqu, RMK, Chanel, Armani and Bobbi Brown, though only the latter two cater properly for darker skins, which is galling. I apply cream foundation with a flat synthetic foundation brush, using the back of my hand as a palette. Creams come in either a pot, stick or a solid compact. My strong preference is in that order too.

Suitable for
Oily, normal or combination skins.
Not suitable for
Mature, dry, dehydrated or dull skins.

You see fewer of these in the noughties, but they still exist. A powder foundation looks like a regular powder compact but the product within has a creamier, waxier texture and a sponge applicator instead of a puff. Powder foundations can be brilliantly convenient for weekends away, holidays or post-gym or pre-evening touch-ups, but they don't give brilliant coverage and can look patchy on the wrong skin types. Applied properly and appropriately, though, a powder foundation can give a subtle, light coverage and a sort of polished, smart look to the face. My favourites are by Stila, Clinique, Guerlain, Givenchy and MAC.

HOW TO FIND YOUR
PERFECT FOUNDATION SHADE

When you have decided which formula is for you, then it's time to find your perfect shade. Some on-counter staff are much better than others at colour matching, so the right foundation can be a lottery. This is the way to perfectly colour match, whether your skin is as white as flour or as black as carbon.

The vast majority of women look prettier in a yellow-based foundation, as opposed to a pink one, whatever their skin tone. You know how pretty you look in a restaurant, bathed in candlelight? That's the yellowy gold flattering your skin. Pink makes you look embalmed or consumptive. There are probably only five women in every hundred who are so extremely pale that they need a pink-toned foundation. Everyone else: if you see pink in the shade, or come across any foundation with the word rose in the colour name, avoid it like the plague. Frankly, I'd rather have pink hair than a pink foundation. Keep pink confined to lips, cheeks and nails, where it belongs.

To choose a colour, look at the section of a brand's shade spectrum you think, by sight, your complexion inhabits, avoiding any pinks unless you are alabaster-white. Take three or four foundation samples in that section and apply them, one next to the other, in small but obvious stripes across your lower cheek. Don't blend.

Repeat the process on your forehead. This can often need a different shade, especially for women of colour, who sometimes need two foundations.

Go outside. You will look daft but not half as silly as if wearing a crap foundation later. Department-store lighting can be at best unrepresentative and at worst woeful (yes, Debenhams, I am looking at you). A look at your face in daylight will give you a much more realistic idea of how a colour looks in real life.

Hold a hand mirror at arm's length and look at your face. One of the stripes will be very hard to see. You may need to squint to see its outline. That is your foundation.

Do not be tempted to try to 'correct' what you perceive to be faults in your skin tone by going up or down a shade. The right foundation is the same colour as your skin. It is not there to give it added warmth (this is the job of bronzer), or coolness (this can be done with highlighter). It is there to match perfectly.

Remember that you may need a different foundation according to the time of the year. Many women quickly become much darker in the summer.

Don't be put off if this sounds like a bit of a ball-ache. I haven't had to do this in years – I can now immediately spot my shade from a cursory glance at a tester stand, or sometimes even an online swatch. Identifying a proper colour match becomes second nature as years go on.

Don't rely on smartphone apps that claim to effectively colour match you to the right foundation. As these require your existing foundation shade name to make the match, they can only hope to work if you have previously been perfectly matched and are now looking simply to switch to another brand.

To prime or not to prime?

Most women seem to have little idea about what primer actually is, and I'm not surprised, since it seems to be marketed opaquely, as if anyone needing to ask questions probably shouldn't buy it. But primer is utterly brilliant stuff and not just for the experts.

If you have bumpiness from old acne scars, or you still suffer from rosacea or pimples, if you are going through the menopause and find your make-up runs for cover at the hint of a hot flash, if you're so oily you can't hang on to your make-up beyond elevenses, if your foundation becomes patchy and gathers around random hotspots on your face, or if it sinks into pores and sits there until bedtime – primer is your friend. I wear it whenever I wear foundation and even when I'm not, with just a little concealer and face powder on top.

I am in my late thirties and prone to dullness, so I use a primer with light reflectors to mimic a natural glow, but there are primers for every specific skin problem, from colour corrective versions for uneven tone, to mineral primers for sensitive skins. In every case, what good primers do is sort of 'laminate' your skin with safe silicones, falsely creating a much smoother surface. Foundation coats more evenly and stays there for longer. Ditto concealer and blush, and they are a doss to apply. After your moisturiser, squeeze a pea-sized amount onto the back of your hand and, using your middle fingertip, smooth over your entire face, including your eyelids. Never rub or massage – this can cause silicone to break down and disintegrate into maddening tiny bobbles. When finished, wait a few moments then apply make-up as normal.

The best primers are by Laura Mercier, Smashbox, Dior, Revlon, Illamasqua, Eve Lom, Clinique and Estée Lauder.

How to apply foundation

You can use a sponge, a brush or just fingertips to apply foundation – all are fine, though my preference is a flat synthetic brush. Whichever you opt for, put some foundation on the back of your hand and dot or stroke it onto your face – on the forehead, upper cheeks, jawline, nose, eyelids and chin (or just where you need it if you are blessed with great skin). Then blend together out towards your hair and jawline. If you can see brush or sponge marks in the foundation, you're applying too much of it. You do not need to apply it to your neck – it will ruin your clothes and feel gross. Just blend extra well at the jawline. Follow with concealer to cover any blemishes poking through, and a face powder to set the whole thing.

Freckles

Freckles are the prettiest thing in the world and should never be covered (heavy foundation turns them grey). If you're blessed with freckles, opt for a sheer coverage foundation to show them off. If you also have any uneven tone, spots or blemishes, patch-cover those with concealer (see Basic Kit), not base.

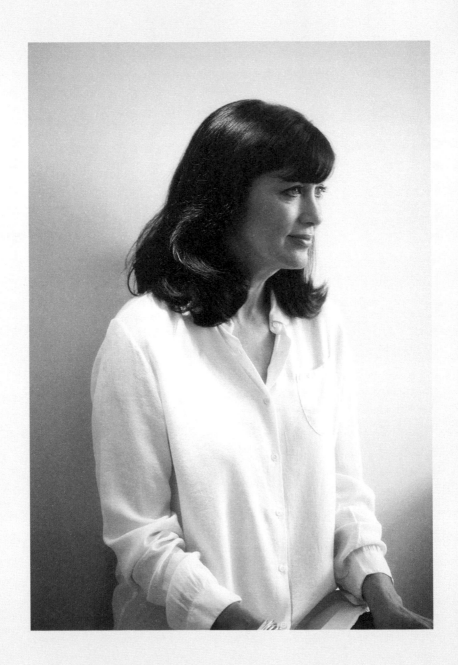

ANTI-AGEING

'Nature gives you the face you have at twenty;
it is up to you to merit the face you have at fifty.'
Coco Chanel

At 39, I am gradually observing first-hand how Beauty's biggest moneyspinner, 'anti-ageing', is made far more complicated than it should be. Millions of slightly baffled women are buying into impossible technology and cod science at huge personal expense. There are so many different products and so many assertions made that even as I attempt to communicate the basics here, I'm almost wincing in anticipation of incurring the wrath of those in my industry with vastly different points of view from my own.

But anyway, here, in brief, is what happens to the skin as we age. Your skin has three layers. The surface layer is called the epidermis, the second, the dermis. Finally, the deepest layer is called the hypodermis. The epidermis is what we see, and bears the visual hallmarks of the condition of the dermis beneath – sunspots, lines, ill health and so on. The dermis is the really important layer in terms of beauty, not only because its condition determines how the ground level looks, but because as well as producing sebaceous (oil-making) glands to keep the surface moist, it is composed largely of collagen (which makes skin plump) and elastin (making it stretchy, supple and elastic). These proteins are abundant in young skin and give it its gorgeous appearance. Annoyingly, these proteins naturally diminish as we age – faster if we smoke or overexpose ourselves to the sun. The deep hypodermis layer contains the functional stuff – veins, nerve, blood vessels and so on. Think of skin as a television set: the epidermis is the screen we watch; the dermis, the inner mechanics that directly affect the picture; and the hypodermis is the cable and plug that allows the whole thing to function in the first place.

So can we slow the progress of these diminishing proteins with anti-ageing skincare ingredients? Before I answer that, I need to define exactly what I mean by anti-ageing. There are many, many ingredients – both natural and chemical – that I fully believe help skin look much better. But that is not the same as believing that they slow the skin's natural ageing process. When it comes to any skincare, it really depends how you define 'effective'. There is, frankly, a great deal to recommend, say, a face cream that smells nice, provides a smooth base for make-up, makes skin feel comfortable, moist and supple, look fresh and dewy and generally in great nick at any age. That is not an anti-ageing product, it's a great moisturiser and everyone should own one. An anti-ageing cream, however, sets its sights higher still; it also promises to slow the ageing process, to prevent the lines, discolouration and loss of volume that are entirely natural in all human faces as they get older. Anti-ageing skincare is controversial because it both implies there's something inherently wrong with looking one's age and at the same time promises to perform a feat that seems highly unlikely.

It's unlikely for one huge reason, from my lay perspective: beauty brands (and let's face it, we) are preoccupied with the (upper) epidermis and yet we know the best way to make real differences to the ageing process is to treat the condition of what lies beneath it in the dermis. The fundamental problem with this is that the skin is designed to form a protective barrier that doesn't welcome strangers through the front door, so to speak. It's there to protect us. In other words, topical skincare products cannot get to where they want to go, into the dermis, to deliver their hi-tech anti-ageing ingredients.

How does this affect you? Well, brands will tell you all the time that their new cream or serum contains proven anti-ageing ingredients and they are very often right. What they have so far been largely unable to prove (again, to me) is that these ingredients will ever get the chance to work. It's all very well injecting ingredients into deeper skin cells sitting in a petri dish then marvelling at their favourable reaction, but in practice, they will only ever be smeared onto the epidermis by consumers in their bathrooms. Rest assured, the skincare industry is obsessed with overcoming this fundamental problem (which seems impossible, but so did most medical advances at the time of breakthrough) and spends literally billions on the very best scientific research, correct in the knowledge that we will all buy the product that finally nails it. (Incidentally, the 'evil beauty industry' so many enjoy vilifying happens to be paying for countless potentially life-saving medical research projects worldwide, in the hope they will also yield breakthroughs in anti-ageing skincare. Potential unlimited profits for them, sure, but also pretty important for everyone, so let's not be ignorant to its beneficial by-products.)

So, those are the basics, which may depress you or confirm your existing suspicions, or both. That moisturiser on which you spent £100 may feel great and look lovely, but it is not going to fix your jowls or put your eyelids back up where they once lived. That said, it is not all doom and gloom. There are a small handful of lifestyle choices and, yes, skincare ingredients, that have been proven to make real improvements to ageing skin (or slow the signs), as well as a few that are increasingly looking as though they very well may do something interesting (there are many of them and a mountain of research available online, should you be interested in reading more. Be prepared for conflicting opinion). I have separated both kinds clearly below.

THINGS WE KNOW WORK

NOT SMOKING

Smokers ultimately look older than non-smokers. This is just a fact. If you're not convinced, walk through town and look at anyone standing outside a pub or restaurant. Imagine them without the cigarette in their hand, look at their faces, and ask yourself if you would still know they were smokers. Nine times out of ten, the answer will be yes. The cloud of smoke around you, whether you stand outside or in (and whether you can see it or not) is attacking your skin's collagen and elastin fibres with toxins. It will make your skin less bouncy, less bright, more vulnerable to dryness, dehydration and deep wrinkles. Your mouth will develop fine lines and lose volume from all that slight puckering up. You may smoke now and be unable to see it (I've been there myself) but I promise you will see the damage later and regret carrying on for so long. Get help from your doctor and quit. Your face will thank you for it.

HYALURONIC ACID

Hyaluronic acid sounds scary but it is, in fact, an entirely natural substance already present in the body. Its cleverness is in its ability to hold more than a thousand times its own weight in water. The cosmetic effect of this is akin to soaking a raisin in a glass of water – the surface of the skin looks plumper, fatter, smoother, younger. It has proven long-term benefits when injected into the skin, but back in the real world, it still significantly improves the appearance of skin when applied topically. It's also pretty cheap and is widely used in serums, creams, foundations, lip balms and body lotions and can be used on any skin type, even very oily or sensitive, at any age. I cannot recommend it enough – it makes an instant and noticeable difference. Check for sodium hyaluronate in your ingredients list. It should be in the first seven listed ingredients for a good concentration (it will never be the first or second, so don't drive yourself crazy looking for it).

RETINOL

Retinoids – either in the form of Retin-A from a doctor, or in consumer beauty products – are a form of vitamin A, and are the best, and indeed, only, topical treatment we have for long-term reduction in wrinkles and other sun damage (retinoids are also prescribed for acne, psoriasis and even skin cancers). Retinol creams typically reduce pores, too. A 2008 study by the University of Michigan found that topical retinol application was one of only three proven treatments for ageing skin (the other two were carbon dioxide laser treatments and hyaluronic acid injections, both administered by a cosmetic practitioner [source: Singer]). Retinol is not cheap (you're unlikely to get a decent retinol cream for less than about £18) and not the gentlest ingredient. It sometimes causes flaking and redness (especially when prescription strength) though rarely for more than a week. Over time, retinol (usually delivered in cream form) can fade age spots and noticeably reduce wrinkles and other sun damage. Retinol products must always be used in conjunction with a broad-spectrum sunblock, as the ingredient leaves skin more vulnerable to sun damage. For more on retinols, see the chapter on acne.

EXERCISE

The case for regular exercise is pretty clear. Those who do it typically live longer and are slower to show signs of ageing. They are likely to retain higher muscle mass, stronger bones and better health overall. Given that the outer appearance of our skin is a visible indicator of the health of its lower layers, then the connection between healthy body and good-looking skin is a pretty clear one. On a more specific and anecdotal level, I personally hold a great deal of stock in facial massage. It seems entirely sensible to me that when the structure of your face is formed by muscle, which is also propping up skin, you do your bit to keep those muscles in shape. If choosing a facial in a salon, my advice is to not be too steered by brand or product, but to book one that focuses on massage – those are usually the best and more long lasting in effect (my skin seems firmer and looks brighter for at least a week). Facial exercise is important too. Five minutes' facial exercise at home, in front of the telly or during your morning routine has, in my view, a noticeable effect. There are lots of good tutorials on YouTube and some good tools like facial massage rollers are available on the high street.

AHAs

Alpha Hydroxy Acids treat the surface of the skin to impressive effect, very often giving it a noticeably younger-looking and more vibrant appearance. These acids basically gobble up dead skin cells that make older skin in particular seem lacking in vibrancy. They also help spots, enlarged and clogged pores and strip away the cells collected around, and exacerbating the appearance of, fine lines. AHAs are very helpful but, unlike hyaluronates (see above), are not to be used abundantly and without consideration. They are to be used between one and four times a week, depending on the concentration of your AHA solution (liquids will typically be higher than creams). Sensitive skins are best suited to a lower concentration of around 3 per cent, while more hardy types may be able to take something of around 5 per cent twice a week. Follow the manufacturer's instructions carefully and never, ever use AHAs without applying sunscreen before leaving the house.

This is absolutely essential as newly exposed skin cells will be more susceptible to irritation and long-term damage.

SUNSCREEN

Long-term UVA and UVB exposure (or one-off overexposure) attacks collagen and elastin fibres and ages the skin. It also commonly causes unevenness in skin tone, and contrary to popular belief, is broadly indiscriminate towards natural skin colour. One of the most important things you can do for your skin is protect it with a broad-spectrum sunscreen (protecting against both UVB that more commonly causes burning and skin cancers, as well as UVA, more usually responsible for premature skin ageing) with an SPF of 15 or more, whenever you expose your skin to extended periods in sunlight. I say extended because some level of vitamin D obtained from sunlight is important to physical health. I might not wear an SPF to nip out for a paper or to drop off my kids at school, but I would never eat lunch outside, or walk the dog, without one. Use your common sense. When in strong sunlight (i.e. during spring and summer or when visiting sunny climes), I recommend wearing an SPF of at least 30 whenever outside, and buying a hat. And always protect your children. A shocking amount of sun damage is caused during childhood, the results of which cannot be seen for decades.

Some of the things we think may work

Antioxidants

Antioxidants are substances thought to protect cells from the damage caused by free radicals (aggressors that break down collagen and elastin, including cigarette smoke, pollution, etc) in our everyday environments. We ingest antioxidants through our food and know some of them to be helpful. What we don't know is whether or not they do the same good work when applied to the surface of the skin. Certainly, the vast majority of cosmetic dermatologists I meet believe in antioxidants and prescribe them widely, and purely on an anecdotal level, very many women (including practically all beauty editors) believe they improve the look and feel of their skin. Some clinical studies concur, some don't. The dermatology community seems divided. I use serums and creams with antioxidants like an agnostic prays – they do me no harm and, well, you never know...

Vitamin C

Vitamin C is an antioxidant (see above), but its status as an effective anti-ageing ingredient is now so recognised that it is a little further ahead in the race, especially when taken through food. It's loved by many cosmetic dermatologists for its connection to healthy collagen production, perceived 'glow-giving' benefits and its beneficial effect on sunburn. But there are some key scientists who disagree that enough clinical evidence bears this out. Vitamin C appears in lots of anti-ageing serum and cream ingredients lists and in beauty supplements and that can only be a good thing, but the best way of ensuring its benefits is to take it internally as food.

Good nutrition

Few things divide skincare experts like nutrition. Many cosmetic dermatologists (whether in private practice or as brand consultants) will point out that there is no decisive evidence that a healthy, nutritious and balanced diet has any effect on the skin's ageing process, and yet in my personal experience they also routinely counsel against eating too much sugar because they believe it to accelerate it. They almost always prescribe the intake of essential fatty acids and fish oils (no one can tell me these don't improve skin). As a layperson, this strikes me as somewhat confusing and contradictory – if a diet too high in sugar can adversely affect the ageing process, then I am happy to presume that a healthy diet can be beneficial to it. Certainly, I believe my own skin reacts badly to too much sugar (it's only ever spotty at Christmas, when my sugar consumption is at an annual high, to name but one example) and looks well when I've been eating plenty of fresh produce. I also feel that given how much expert support there now is for vitamin C (see above) as an anti-ageing ingredient in skincare, then surely a good intake of vitamin C in our diets is potentially even better?

FAST FIXES

If anti-ageing skincare seems too vague, too expensive, too much like hard work, then these tricks will knock years off in a flash.

GET A FRINGE

Fringes are youthful, cute and are easily the most effective alternative to Botox on forehead lines. Ten minutes at the hairdresser's (never cut one in yourself) and they're hidden from view.

PINCH YOUR CHEEKS

A trick as old as time and one that works. Pinching your cheeks lightly gets blood flowing to the face, restoring a little glow and giving the skin a youthful-looking flush.

USE AN EXFOLIATING MASK

Good exfoliating masks usually work in just a couple of minutes to rid the skin of dead surface cells that make it look older and more tired.

Stroke a smooth (no grains), creamy exfoliating mask over a dry face. Wait for the allocated time (usually between one and five minutes) and loosen the mask with water. Remove what remains with a wrung-out warm flannel. Follow with something moisturising like an oil or cream.

APPLY PINK BLUSH

Everyone looks a little younger with a little pink in their cheeks – it's almost the most flattering thing one can easily do with make-up. Pink blush suits everyone of every age and colour and comes in a finish for every skin type too. If you like easy finger application, go for creme or gel formulas, if you're reasonably adept at make-up, choose powder. Whichever you wear, pop it just on the apples of the cheeks to mimic a natural, youthful flush.

CURL YOUR LASHES

Curling your lashes makes eyes appear instantly uplifted and more awake. Buy a decent set of curlers – spending over ten pounds makes quite a big difference to quality. Looking down into a mirror, clamp on the curlers and ensure you haven't pinched any skin before gently pressing the plates together. Apply mascara. When it's dry, repeat the curling for a stronger and more lasting effect.

GO FOR A BRISK WALK

A brisk walk in the open air gets the circulation going and makes dull skin look more awake and vibrant. I strongly believe that everyone looks better after gentle outdoor exercise.

APPLY BODY MAKE-UP

You really need not tolerate the visible veins, cellulite and uneven tone associated with ageing skin on your limbs. Body make-up and wash-off tans are now brilliantly easy, blend well and don't transfer onto your clothes. Even easier are gradual-tanning body lotions you just slather on after showering to conceal a multitude of minor imperfections.

My own daily skincare products

The brands change a lot, but the key ingredients
and principles remain much the same. This is what
I will typically use in a day:

A cream or balm cleanser containing plant oils
and no particular 'anti-ageing' ingredients.

....

An AHA liquid exfoliant (2–3 times a week).

....

An anti-ageing serum containing hyaluronic acid
and antioxidants, including vitamin C.

....

An anti-ageing day cream containing hyaluronic acid, antioxidants
and an SPF20 (a total sunblock in spring and summer).

....

A natural plant facial oil, followed by an anti-ageing night
cream containing hyaluronic acid and retinol.

....

A lip balm containing hyaluronic acid.

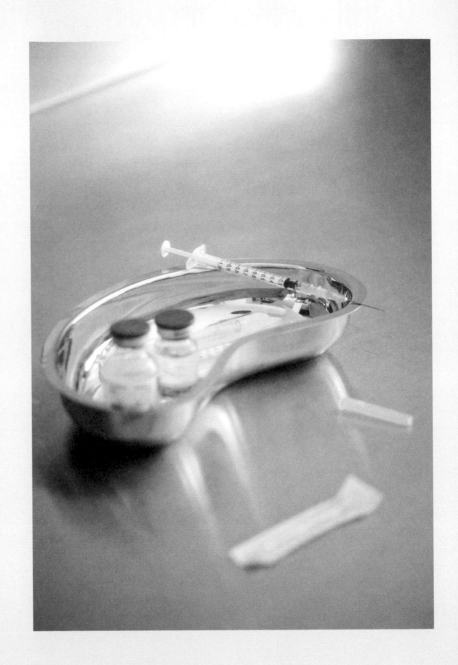

HOW TO GET BOTOX

'Beauty without expression is boring.'
Ralph Waldo Emerson

Few beauty issues divide women more than that of Botox, the 'anti-ageing' injections made into the face, hands and neck to literally paralyse tiny muscles that exacerbate the appearance of wrinkles.

I have no problem whatsoever with a principled objection to putting Botox in one's own face. I accept and broadly agree with many of the very valid concerns that women are under more pressure than ever to look younger than their years in order to be valued, and at often great financial cost. I positively admire those who make a stand and opt out, just as I respect those who choose of their own free will to go ahead.

But I also feel very strongly that it's perfectly natural to want to look as youthful as we now behave, live and feel inside. Senior women nowadays are simply not the cauliflower-haired pensioners of yore. There's nothing wrong with not wanting to look knackered when you are, in fact, full of energy. I see no problem with seeking to restore the natural glow present in our twenties and thirties, even if that means cheating a little. It seems perfectly reasonable to want your brows to stay up where they were and not gatecrashing your eyelids, or to decide that that one deep crease between your eyes is really bloody annoying and can bugger off for the cost of a new coat. This is where Botox and fillers can be enormously helpful.

And while I understand the political reasons for avoiding Botox, people's more commonly held aversions on grounds of aesthetics do slightly get my goat. Everyone seems to have an opinion on the appearance of Botox, which I find very interesting, given that very few seem to know what it really looks like. They will cite examples like Joan Rivers, David Gest, reality TV stars who positively delight in looking like startled tambourines. But the irony is that those who say women with Botox look mad are by definition talking about the bad and excessive Botox you can identify at 100 paces. No one can criticise and laugh at the good stuff because when Botox is administered correctly and in moderation, it is undetectable even to my trained eye, and can look absolutely brilliant. Botox can imperceptibly remove a deep frown line, making you appear to have been on a six-week holiday. It can smooth away eye wrinkles and stop your eyes drooping downwards in a way that suggests you've had your first good night's sleep in years.

Good Botox can basically make you feel like yourself while everyone else is none the wiser.

Nonetheless, I see women in my professional and social circles who frankly need to lay the hell off the injectables STAT. There are three looks: 'old', 'young' and 'done', and many women I meet most definitely fall into the latter camp. Their faces are expressionless, frozen in time, too plump, too pillowy, too taut, too bloody surprised, leaving the beholder to assume suspiciously that someone who is probably a perfectly healthy 40-something is, in fact, ancient and desperately ashamed of it. When this occurs, the problem is usually one or both of the following: a crap practitioner, or not waiting until the last dose has worn off before having another one. Both are woefully common.

Finding a good doctor is absolutely key to getting a good and, most importantly, safe result. Your GP will know of good cosmetic doctors. Comparing notes with other women on a beauty forum is also a good way to perform your due diligence. As a general rule, I would not personally visit any plastic or cosmetic surgeon who hasn't done at least a substantial chunk of time working within the NHS or an overseas public health service equivalent, and I'd always expect to see lots of pictures of former patients either on a website or in albums at the clinic. I would reject any treatment whereby my consultation was with anyone other than the person treating me.

An experienced Botox practitioner, whether a cosmetic dermatologist or plastic surgeon, will look carefully at your face and err on the side of caution. S/he will use a weak dilute of Botox and inject very small amounts into several tiny sites, rather than jack up a large area in one shot (this second way is what causes that Ming the Merciless brow look). This will cause only minor discomfort and will heal very soon after. S/he will not start writing a shopping list of other things that need 'fixing' on your face and she will tell you not to come back for more within a three-month (minimum) period. No one should ever 'top up' Botox until it has completely worn off and things have returned to normal. Make an appointment in anticipation of this, by all means, but don't go near a clinic while your previous treatment is in effect. The same applies to fillers. No one tells you this but trust me, people who don't do this look weird. I've stared at heaps of them. They cannot go even a day without effective Botox and impatiently overlap treatments to the detriment of their face. Every three, or more likely six, months is plenty.

I'm stunned by how cavalier women have become about Botox, nipping into hair salons for a top-up or, God forbid, attending Botox parties to pick at a cheese and pineapple hedgehog while they wait to be shot in the forehead with botulism. I would never get Botox or any other quasi-medical cosmetic procedure in a hair salon, chiropodist or optician (yes, really, this exists), beauty salon, high-street skin clinic, shopping centre (I am practically sobbing as I type), any hen party setting or via an overseas cosmetic surgery holiday (I am sick to death of the British health service picking up the tab for overseas botch jobs on people who scrimped on their own faces). You would not let a stranger in the street pierce your ears, let alone inject your face with poison. Putting a shop front between you and them, give or take a short training course, barely changes things. This is your face, for heaven's sake. You get only one. Show it some respect.

GET A TALKING MIRROR FRIEND

Before you go near a doctor, it's imperative that you choose a talking mirror friend. This is a close friend who can be absolutely honest with you about any Botox, fillers or surgery without fear of offending you, whose opinion you trust and take on board. This is the friend who must have the courage to say, 'You're starting to look strange, enough now, darling; stop it, they're only wrinkles, let's have a gin instead'. She will act as your talking mirror to stop you losing sight of how you look (so easily done), who will pull rank on you if you fall into the 'I'll just get one more thing fixed...' trap. I know that if my time comes, my talking mirror is my friend India because she will tell me to chill out and I'll know she's right and will listen. Do not embark on Botox, fillers or anything else involving needles without your own talking mirror. It is utterly essential.

What is Botox and what does it do?

Botulinum toxin is a protein and neurotoxin produced
by the bacterium Clostridium botulinum (the most
acutely toxic substance known). In beauty applications,
it is injected in minute quantities into overactive muscles
to weaken them and reduce movement. This, in turn,
reduces the appearance of fine expression lines around the
eyes, forehead and mouth. The effect will generally take around
48 hours to kick in and last between three and six months.

....

Botox is largely ineffective on deep, established
wrinkles caused by sagging. These sorts of lines are
commonly treated with fillers, which use injections of
harmless substances like hyaluronic acid to add volume,
literally plumping out the skin. In my experience, they
have a more distinctive appearance than Botox, and are
consequently easier to spot.

....

You can expect good Botox to cost £200–250 per site,
e.g. forehead (a treatment costing this is not an indicator
of a good practitioner, you must still do your homework);
£100 or less is too cheap. Save up or leave it. Don't go there.

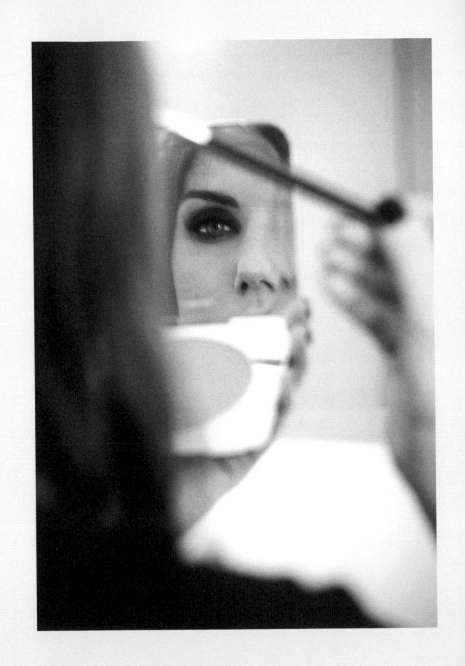

BROWS

'You must never underestimate the power of the eyebrow.'
Jack Black

Well-shaped eyebrows will change your face more dramatically than any product ever could. They sit there, quietly being the most important feature on your entire face, while everyone obsesses over the more showboating eyes and lips. When shaped well, brows act as an optical illusion, opening up eyes and making them appear more awake, your face more perky and alert, even when you're wearing no other make-up. Properly groomed, they make you look chic, elegant, grown up and pulled together. They're extremely helpful when you want to give children or colleagues a terrifying and furious expression. They make applying eyeshadow much easier because they give more space, shape and structure to the entire eyelid, especially when your lids are hooded. They add interest against spectacles. Brows are the frames to your entire face. To painstakingly make up the rest and ignore them is to shove a Helmut Newton in an Ikea clip frame. If you ignore your brows you are missing a trick. Look at any beautiful woman of the past – old or young, blonde or brunette, black or white, siren or gamine – and I can almost guarantee she has a brilliant pair of brows. They are, to me, the key to good grooming.

My brows are my best feature and yet still, like a ninny, I plucked them to practically nothing as a teen in the nineties, in some homage to Linda Evangelista on the cover of *Vogue* – I'm pretty sure a beret was also involved, and some fishnets. I stood in front of a full-length mirror (not even a magnifying one!) before a night out at the pub and plucked away like some starving bird picking worms from the soil. My saving grace was that I took nothing from above the arch, only from under it. This preserved the natural shape and saved me. Nonetheless, they were so thin that my face looked absolutely massive for the next five years, as though someone had drawn some features on a wooden spoon with a Sharpie.

Nowadays, my brows are expertly threaded by the great Daxita Vaghela of Atherton Cox, London. I believe wholeheartedly in the ancient art of brow threading, where a practitioner winds thread around her fingers, holding it taut between her teeth, and removes any stray brow hairs (including those tiny, fuzzy blonde ones) quickly and precisely, row by row, while you hold your eyelid down. It is painful for some, at least at first (it definitely becomes much less so after multiple treatments) but I personally find it to be broadly fine. It does make me sneeze, though, and I can't do anything public for two hours after as I am fairly red.

In any case, a good thread will yield by far the best-looking brow shape – sharp, precise, elegant and clean, but like anything, it must be in the right hands. You can pay anything up to £40 for a brow thread, but cost is by no means a signifier of quality. I've seen some brilliant brows that cost a fiver and some terrible ones at £30 and, of course, vice versa. What's most important is that you seek a personal recommendation. A safe-ish starting point is to seek out a practitioner from a culture in which the revered art of threading is passed from mother to daughter (my own brow guru Daxita was taught by her grandmother to thread at just eleven years old, and has been honing her craft ever since). Communities with a high Asian population are likely to have very experienced threaders locally. When it comes to threading, a two-day cram-course is simply not going to cut it. Brows are simply too important to hand over to someone who doesn't understand that they need to be perfect. Also, I would rather die than obtain a brow thread – or indeed any beauty treatment – in an open kiosk in the middle of a shopping centre. It is madness. Some mystery and decorum, people, please.

If for any reason you decide against threading, tweeze instead. Make a one-off professional appointment to get the initial shape put in, then invest £20 or so in an excellent pair of tweezers (Rubis make the best) to maintain them. You will need to pluck stray hairs outside the immediate area to keep everything neat. Plucking immediately after showering, when pores are temporarily open, minimises pain, as does necking a Nurofen 20 minutes before, but anyone will find that over time both become unnecessary. Always pluck from below, never from the upper half of the brow. You should only ever head north to pluck brow hairs migrating up your temples or between your brows. Don't even think about waxing brows; it's not so much painful as woefully unpredictable and imprecise and can cause ingrown hairs.

Brows that have left the building

It is a horrible thing, when you've overplucked your brows for so long that they take their ball home in a huff and refuse to come back. Most youthful indiscretions can be forgotten, but bald brows are a cruel reminder of earlier stupidity. My whole face changed when I grew mine back from over-plucked hell. It was a slog, but so worth it. If you've been over zealous, here's how to restore yours.

Buy some brow growth serum like Rapid Brow or Talika.
It's expensive and a bore (it must be applied every night
without fail), but it works in many cases. You should see
increased growth in around six weeks.

....

Let them grow. This may be stating the obvious but it's alarming
how many women continue to pluck brows they're already unhappy
with. I understand they will look a mess for a while, but it's a question
of pushing through the pain barrier. They'll look untidy for no more
than a month (starting the process before a holiday helps) and you can
keep them looking half decent with clear brow gel. Put up with it now
and you'll have laid the groundwork for a lifetime of good brows.

....

When brows have grown through (possibly patchily), see a
professional threader and get them properly shaped, even if you
have not the time, cash nor inclination to continue long term.
A professional shape is much easier to follow with tweezers
at home. Consider also having your brows tinted, as sparse
brows look more substantial when darker.

....

If nothing works, and brows fail to grow back, consider
semi-permanent brow resurrection. (See tattooed brows.)

....

Fill in whenever you make-up. (See following pages.)

Tattooed brows

Tattooed-on brows can offer a great solution to women who've permanently lost their brows from overplucking, alopecia or chemotherapy, but it's absolutely essential you put in the time and money to get the best practitioner, and only do this when you've tried in earnest to grow back your natural brows. A good brow tattooist will have an album of his/her work and usually some personal testimonials from former clients. Many chemotherapy staff will be able to recommend someone nearby too.

Personally speaking, I think the most impressive solution is via Browhaus' Brow Resurrection service, a semi-permanent solution lasting around three years. Instead of tattooing on a brow shape, as other practitioners do (with wildly varying degrees of success), Browhaus tattoo on each and every hair individually, tapering it at the end for an astonishingly natural result. The technique can be used on non-existent or just sparse brows of any colour, and must be re-done to refresh every few years. It is worth the cash and hassle – they fool almost everybody.

A NOTE ON COLOUR

Brows are not warm and I wish beauty brands would wake up to the fact. However warm your hair and skin colour, your brows will almost certainly be a cold, flat colour somewhere between 'dirty dishwater' and 'oily puddle' – and that works perfectly. A warm brow pencil or powder immediately looks dyed and wiggy. I personally love how dark brown brows look on everyone, from pale blonde (very Hitchcock heroine) to silver (brows cost practically nothing to dye and look so chic against grey), but your mileage may vary. The important thing is that your chosen colour is convincingly cool-toned. Blondes and greys look good in grey-taupe, redheads suit flat, murky grey-browns and brunettes can wear anything from muddy brown to ashy black. All can be filled in at a pinch with a common or garden graphite school pencil, which tends to look natural on everyone and comes off easily with cleansing milk (they haven't contained lead in decades, in case you're panicking).

How to fill in brows

I don't fill in my brows every day, but I would never neglect to if wearing a full make-up. A little colour allows them to remain holding court when your face is bustling with other products, and adds a great deal of elegance. I will happily gambol about my daily business with only a little clear brow gel or Vaseline (or even nothing), but just as I feel about heeled shoes, I would never attend a meeting without my game-brows on. Here's how I do it.

After applying base (foundation, concealer and powder), comb brows into shape with an old, dry mascara wand. Comb upwards until you hit your natural arch, then stroke downwards beyond it.

....

Take a stiff, angled synthetic brush – it needs to be short and stubby with no flexibility – and stroke it in some cold-toned, matte brow powder. You will only need a little and can always add more later.

....

Bend your little finger against your cheek as an anchor and, pivoting your hand (not moving your arm at all), stroke along the brow hairs, in the same direction as growth. Your strokes should be short and feathery.

....

Stop at the peak of your natural arch and start stroking downwards in longer, firmer strokes. Check for symmetry.

....

Leave for a few moments then set with brow gel or clear mascara. This should be the cheapest one you can find – it's only hair gel in a mascara wand and anything over a fiver, max, is a waste of money. All brow gels are disgusting-looking within six weeks and need to be binned.

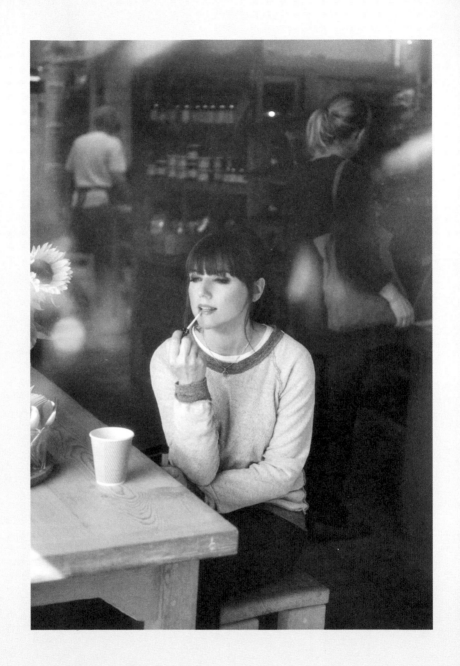

PUBLIC DISPLAYS OF GROOMING

'We never really grow up, we only learn how to act in public.'
Bryan White

I'm writing this on a commuter train from Brighton to London. Before I opened my laptop, I took ten minutes out of my journey to put on some make-up for my lunch meeting in town. Concealer, powder, mascara, blush and lipstick, all applied in my train seat while my fellow passengers did their own thing and failed to bat an eyelid at mine. The woman adjacent to me is tapping away on her computer. The man in front is playing with his iPhone (with keytones switched on, for goodness' sake. There is simply no need.) while the man next to him is listening to YouTube clips through his headphones. No one is doing anyone any harm, including me.

I often apply make-up on the train. It passes the journey time, allows me to get up not quite so early and ensures I look fresh on arrival. I'm never anti-social, because when it comes to public grooming, I have a few unshakeable rules. Nothing that involves shedding – hairbrushing, filing, tweezing, powder puffing (I was once completely appalled to see a woman clipping her nails on the train) – is forgivable; and nothing smelly like nail polish or perfume – I don't think it's okay to subject fellow passengers to your fumes, any more than it's fine to smoke or tuck into some egg sandwiches. Manners are important. I never invade someone's personal space and also tend not to make up if I'm in a facing seat or standing up – it makes me self-conscious and, I imagine, some other passengers uncomfortable. But some simple, discreet make-up application – why not? I can't see the problem. It's not disrupting anyone's journey and I really don't see it as anyone's business.

I will apply lipstick at a restaurant table, and powder my nose in a pub rather than visit a grotty loo. I'll do the same in a doctor's surgery waiting room, more on a train or bus. I see public grooming as no worse than watching someone play Words With Friends, or listening to fellow passengers chat. Certainly, it is less annoying than having one's personal space invaded by the flicking of a huge broadsheet newspaper into the eyes, and infinitely less infuriating than having to listen to someone's unnecessary telephone conversation (my pet hate – speaking in hushed, mortified tones, promising to call back later, is what made this country great). But women trying to apply eyeliner in the 30 seconds a train stands still in a platform, or stroke on lipstick between stops on a shaky 38 bus are some of the little rituals that make up the daily commute. I actively enjoy watching, much as it is sometimes difficult for me not to intervene to tell someone their blusher brush is in dire need of a wash, or that they'd look so much better in rose than fuschia. If you are, on the other hand, irrationally offended by them, I say don't look – it's terribly easy not to. And then perhaps turn your attention to the idiot in headphones playing drum 'n' bass way too loud further down the carriage. Now that *is* out of order.

How to do your face on the bus or train

Before leaving the house, it's very much worth applying tinted moisturiser or foundation. This takes very little time but involves a large area, liquids, brushes, elbows and other things that don't seem terribly social. After that, things are pretty easy to do discreetly from a train or bus seat. Just arm yourself with as many products as possible that can be used without lots of brushes and applicators, e.g. pencils, crayons and cremes. You will also need a small magnifying mirror, preferably one that opens flat rather than at a right angle, so you can hold it close to your face.

Dot concealer under eyes, around the nose and over any blemishes. Pat with your ring finger to blend. (45 seconds)

....

Pat a puff in some pressed powder and stroke over your face, including lids and lips. (20 seconds)

....

Dab your ring finger in a creme eyeshadow. Brown, ivory or taupe are ideal as they're easy to apply. Pat your finger onto each eyelid, covering the lower half and stopping just past the eye crease. Move to your cheeks while this sets. (2 minutes)

....

Dab your middle finger in a creme blush. Pat three dots of colour on each cheek, then stroke together in a circular motion. Then, use a clean fingertip to stroke the furthest edge of the circle into a teardrop shape, feathering it outwards. (60 seconds)

....

Take a chunky eye crayon (the best are by Barry M, Charlotte Tilbury and Smashbox) and line the upper and lower lashline. The fatness of the crayon will mean a shaky train or bus won't make the line anything like as wonky. Smudge lightly with your little finger to soften. (2 minutes)

....

Apply mascara during a stop. If you only have a few seconds, do your lower lashes while you're stationary as this is the trickiest part to do on the move. (30–60 seconds)

....

Use a tinted brow gel (Benefit, MAC, Nars and By Terry all make them) to tint and comb your brows upwards into place. (30 seconds)

....

Leave lipstick until you've finished your coffee and are almost at your destination, then apply straight from the stick. Blot with a tissue or napkin before applying a second coat. Check your teeth. (30 seconds)

....

Do not spritz perfume until you're outside.
Brush your hair at the same time.

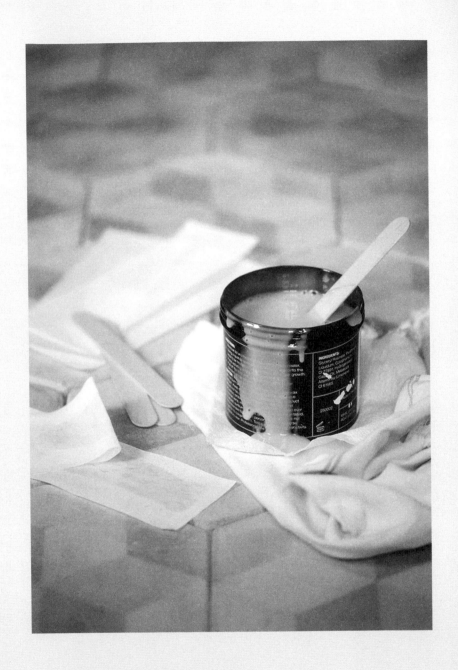

TO WAX OR NOT TO WAX

'I don't understand how a woman can take
boiling hot wax, pour it on upper thighs, rip the
hair out by the roots, and still be afraid of a spider.'
Jerry Seinfeld

Few beauty matters divide feminists more decisively than hair removal, though I am personally conflicted. I too find the widespread adoption of full bikini waxes pretty worrying, and am alarmed by the very real danger that, having digested years of identical pornography and the even more prolific pop videos of young female singers, an entire generation of young people now believes pubic hair to be dirty, abnormal, wholly undesirable or a sign of sloppy grooming. It is no such thing.

But while I am wholly against women feeling they must epilate to conform to society's expectations, I know that in reality there are umpteen other reasons for choosing to do so – from religious beliefs to increased sexual pleasure to sporting activities or just plain personal preference. Sometimes I wax, sometimes I don't, to me, it's just another feature I can experiment with and change when I'm bored. Whatever your reasons – and they should be yours and yours alone – I don't judge. The hypocrisy in this, of course, is that if I meet a man who feels strongly in favour of a cue-ball fronty then I'm afraid I do judge him, and quite harshly (ladies who like a bald scrotum, I'm afraid you make me feel a bit scratchy too). There's something creepy about the thankfully atypical man who has strong views on a woman's vagina (an encouraging but not surprising 2013 study shows that 60 per cent of men don't give a damn). As with every matter of beauty, my distinction is one of female choice, not obligation, and I'm uncomfortable with any man thinking my vagina needs to up its game for anyone. Frankly, having access should be reward enough without my having to mow the lawn in advance of anyone's arrival. There is also the question of infantilism. I'm really not into grown men who are into little girl genitalia. It's creepy and would be enough to make me call a cab and reject any future correspondence.

Of course, while feminism can and probably should intellectualise the issue of waxing ad infinitum, there will always be women to whom only appearances matter. I have no vast problem with this, but feel duty bound to tell them that full Hollywood bikini waxes always make the hips and thighs look bigger. If no other reason compels you to consider your own position, perhaps that will.

How to get a bikini wax

Think carefully about what you want. If you just want a traditional bikini wax that removes hair from either side of your pants when pulled up (a triangle shape, basically), then most beauty salons will be much of a muchness. If you're after a Brazilian (a thin landing strip) or a Hollywood (absolutely everything, even around the back), then you need to choose more carefully. I've had the most atrocious Brazilian that left me looking like a mangy hare, because the therapist, I discovered afterwards, had never before performed one. You need to find a salon that specialises in full waxing – there are even bikini-waxing-only salons open these days, and take some ibuprofen 30 minutes before arriving. The treatment room should be spotless and the therapist wholly unembarrassed (I personally favour a friendly but reassuringly jaded expression).

You will need to leave your dignity at the door, remove your underwear (I take baby wipes for a last-minute freshen up) and steel yourself for legs akimbo action. It will hurt, though less so after repeated treatments. A classic wax takes about 5 minutes, a Brazilian, around 15 and a Hollywood, about 20. The therapist will smooth on aloe gel or something similarly soothing afterwards and tell you not to bath until tomorrow. Any discomfort thereafter should be fleeting. The effect of a bikini wax lasts for around two weeks – four if you're lucky. Do not use a razor in the meantime – the coarse stubble will itch like crazy and in any case, I am broadly against sharp blades hovering anywhere near my clitoris.

EPILATING

Epilating legs, underarms or the face is also a matter of choice, but for me, one far less fraught and laden with gender politics. I think the expectation by both men and women in the real world is fairly easy-going. My legs are mostly shaved (worth it for the orgasmic feeling of just-shaved legs against clean sheets alone), but if they're not, I just pull on my opaques and forget about it. Ditto my underarms, there's not a great deal happening under there and it's not like I'm one of those women who sits around looking fabulous in vest tops anyway. My upper lip and chin I thread for extreme close-up photography (truly, the camera makes everyone look like Frida Kahlo) then I leave it au naturel the rest of the time. Whatever you do and why, there is a perfect method and best practice involved.

I thread my upper lip and chin before every photoshoot (once every two months). This involves a practitioner holding taut a thread between her hands and teeth and pulling it swiftly across the hairs at the root. It makes many women (including me) sneeze like mad, and it's not painless, though this is drastically improved with repeated treatments. You will look red for a couple of hours afterwards. The joy of threading is it's fast, neat, extremely precise and almost never causes ingrown hairs. It's much kinder to skin than waxing, epilation creams and certainly shaving (seriously, you must never do this. What may seem like a convenient emergency measure will fast become the bane of your daily existence), and uses no chemicals, making it ideal for the easily allergic.

Threading lasts a long time – between three and eight weeks, depending on how hirsute the client. If you suffer from coldsores on the threaded area, the act can cause one to appear, so ask the practitioner to dodge the usual hotspots. Some people find they break out in spots on the threaded area, though this can be helped by not putting on rich products or make-up afterwards (I also find sealing the area with aloe gel or a similar barrier product helps a lot). If I can't get a threading appointment, I wax in a salon (but never my brows. Brow waxing is a terrible idea). It's inferior but tolerable.

Legs

If you're epilating large areas like legs, hot waxing has a lot to recommend it. By this I mean the type of waxing that is performed in a salon with either wax and paper strips, or a ball of hot wax rolled over hair growth. Cold wax strips from the chemist are hellish. I once lay in a bath for two hours, practically weeping, trying to ease one off my bush.

Hot wax is spread along the direction of the legs' hair growth, then covered with a paper strip which is removed briskly against the direction of hair growth. This act is repeated all over the area until all the hair is removed. Some therapists bypass the strips altogether and smooth a pliable ball of wax directly onto the hair before removing it.

Waxing is not especially painful – repeated treatments become less so – but many women say it hurts more during ovulation or periods. In any case, it's a good idea to take painkillers 30 minutes before shedding your stockings. Expect results to last 2–6 weeks. Hairs grow back with a natural tapered end, so are less bristly and stubbly than shaving. I don't personally love waxing as I'm annoyed by the downtime as hairs grow long enough to wax again. Ingrown hairs are pretty common too, so I prefer to shave.

HOW TO SHAVE ONE'S LEGS

It seems mad to be telling you something so basic but I know that many women find shaving needlessly blood-shedding, possibly having learnt from a similarly clueless but wise-seeming older girl at school (Zillah Campbell, I'm looking at you). Bad shaving causes pimply, sore, dry legs with nicks. There is simply no need.

Firstly, you must always have a sharp razor and not a disposable one. Blades are infuriatingly expensive but nonetheless, you need them. A good-quality blade will last around five leg shaves. Also, if you are someone who shaves her bikini line, keep a separate razor for the job. Pubic hair is coarser and will blunt the blade faster. Secondly, you need a cream to smooth the surface for the blade to travel along. I like shaving cream, but am just as likely to use a moisturising shower cream like Dove. In extremis, hair conditioner also works, but it is more of a faff to rinse from your razor.

When you get in the shower or bath, drop your razor under the hot water to heat up while you wash your hair. This may sound improbable, but a barber to royalty told me years ago that this gives a better shave and he was absolutely right. Rub in the cream, up and down. Shave against the hair growth in long strokes, bending knees to make your way around the curves. Rinse but take care not to use very hot water, as this causes bumpiness. If you are going to use body scrub, this must always be done beforehand, never afterwards. Do under your arms, if you want to, using the same method. Some people wax here, but I can barely see the point since it takes seconds. Slather the legs in body cream before dressing.

OTHER METHODS

IPL

IPL, or Intense Pulsed Light, is a semi-permanent-to-permanent method of removing hair from anywhere on the body. It can be extremely effective when administered in a salon or by using a good-quality, at-home device made by someone reliable like Phillips or Braun (expensive but good). Either way, it's uncomfortable but not painful and, overall, is one of the epilation methods that is kindest to skin. The problem is that the technology works on colour contrast. This means that black skin with black hair, or white skin with white hair is unresponsive to treatment. The other issue is that, despite many salons offering IPL as a permanent solution, for many, it simply isn't. I've known several cases of women being absolutely delighted with IPL on their bikini line, only to find a year later that everything is back to square one. So it's worth asking yourself whether you're likely to be able to afford to top up. If not, an at-home device would seem more sensible. One thing you should be prepared for: IPL requires you to shave the treated area first. This is understandably the scariest thing about it. But do be reassured that the stubble will be culled in your first treatment and that shaving will not be an ongoing issue. Under no other circumstances but these should you shave your face.

Epilation creams
Veet (formerly Immac) is so, so much better than it used to be. Where it once smelled like perming lotion and stung like agitated wasps, it now does a very effective job without making a nuisance of itself. You stroke on the cream (I find the in-shower foams patchy), leave for ten minutes or so, according to the instructions, then scrape it off with the blunt razor-type gizmo that acts a bit like a squeegy. Where epilation creams fall down is in duration. The effects last a couple of days longer than shaving but nowhere near as long as waxing or threading. The upshot is that, while I know they're now pretty good, I can rarely be bothered with such a faff for relatively little gain.

Plucking
Plucking is good for stray brows and the kind of isolated hairs that invade the post-35-year-old chin – the sort that feel unlike the downy hair on the rest of your face and stand to attention like pipe cleaners. Use super-sharp quality tweezers like Rubis or Tweezerman and remove these stray hairs every day or two.

Epilators
I have never known pain like the time in 1989 when I used my schoolfriend's electric epilator for about half a second on my inner shin. In those days they were like medieval torture implements and I've no idea how anyone tolerated them. Nowadays, they're a fair bit better, though by no means without pain. They work by placing a vibrating metal coil against hair growth which turns, pinches each hair and plucks it out. The effects last as long as waxing (and with the same risk of ingrown hairs), only with the advantage of being able to treat the area again before stubble appears (good epilators, like those by Braun and Phillips, can remove hairs as small as a grain of sand). Their problem is that while similar to waxing in many regards, epilators represent a pain that is self-inflicted. It's instinctively very hard to hold something that really hurts against your own skin, even if waxing by a beauty therapist is a relative walk in the park.

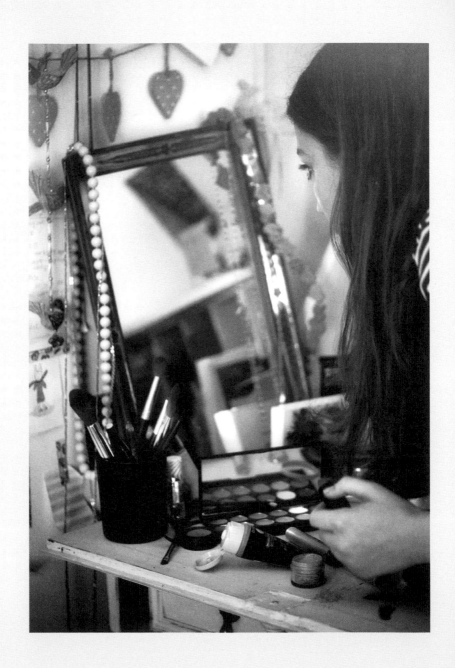

TEEN BEAUTY

'I'm selfish, impatient, and a little insecure. I make
mistakes, I'm out of control, and at times hard to
handle. But if you can't handle me at my worst,
then you sure as hell don't deserve me at my best.'
Marilyn Monroe

Soon after my fifteenth birthday, and very unhappy, I left home with a bag of clothes and a twenty-pound note. My ticket from Hengoed to London cost £12-something. I managed to move in with my then boyfriend and his female flatmate but, too young for anyone to really take me on, I had an employment problem and no money. I'd always done well at school but was still a year away from my exams. I'd never had any intention of becoming anything other than a fashion writer and didn't really know how to do anything else. Except beauty.

My lifelong magazine addiction, childhood under an NHS dermatologist's care and my utter fascination with products and faces had given me a chance at earning some desperately needed money. I was introduced to a well-known London make-up artist of the day, Lynne Easton (known to everyone as 'Pearl', she tragically died in 2005) at Fred's bar in Soho and she asked me to become her assistant. My first job was working on a commercial for Lindt chocolate, helping Pearl to make 40 or so extras look like famous movie stars – Marilyn Monroe, James Dean and so on. My second was on a Pet Shop Boys' video, mattifying Neil Tennant's nose with Shiseido face powder as he sang from a fake courtroom set. It was quite the baptism of fire.

While I learned a truly huge amount working with Pearl, it is still fairly staggering to me that I got through these jobs when I had no real experience. I've come to believe the credit can be laid at the door of an adolescence making make-up mistake after mistake. My mother, though very well groomed and adept herself, never once told me to remove whatever horror I'd plonked on my face that day. She never told me to 'wash that crap off', even when I was wearing roll-on blue eyeshadow and frosty lipstick with Britain's worst-perm since records began. She never said 'You're not going out looking like that...' and so I did.

This sort of freedom is crucial at a time when creativity is so rife and I hope parents realise this. Bonkers or crap make-up is a teenage rite of passage and my past is as littered with disasters as any. From painting lightning bolts down my cheeks with a No17 face-paint set, to becoming addicted to Miss Selfridge copper lipstick that made me look embalmed, to sweet, sickly gloss that made mozzies use my lips as a pitstop, to a mullet haircut frosted with horrible yellow highlights, I have looked as bad as a teenager could. Nonetheless, my teens were the years I learned to love beauty, when I realised how make-up could make my eyes look bigger, my second-hand outfits look better, the beauty mark on my left cheek look cool, not weird. I realised my flat hair could be bigger, curlier, pinker and it would all be back to normal after a bath.

Teenage years are a brilliant time to enjoy beauty because mistakes are not only forgivable, they are crucial. No one is scanning your face with a view to giving you a job, no one is deciding whether to buy your insurance policy or to ask for your hand in marriage. You've no lines, no wrinkles, no visible sun damage, no ingrained habits. Meanwhile, the anxieties of youth – identity issues, creeping insecurity, even problem skin – can all impel you to wear or try something different. It's a great, if not untroubled, basis from which to learn.

And so I hesitate to tell any teenager how they should wear their make-up because I'd slightly hate them to listen to me. There are heaps of general make-up and skincare tips in this book (including an entire chapter on dealing with acne) and they work for every woman, old and young, palest white to darkest black. Read them, try them if you wish, adapt, change and enjoy. It's your face and I implore you to explore it.

A QUICK TEEN FACE

Okay, so I strongly suggest teens go forth and enjoy make-up and not attempt to look like tasteful career women of means, but if you want a quick, easy, adult-friendly face for proms, school graduation, first job interviews, university open days, dates, meeting his parents and the like, then this is how to get it.

Tinted moisturiser
Any without mineral oil are fine. Choose a shade the same colour or only a fraction darker than your skin (unlike foundation, tinted moisturiser is sheer and natural-looking enough to go a fraction darker if you wish). Dot some onto your nose, cheeks, chin and forehead and blend in with fingers. I beg of you, do not opt for foundation here instead. Concealer better covers spots without masking your natural prettiness.

Concealer
Choose a concealer the same colour as your skin, or a fraction lighter. A thick one with some light reflectors is perfect. Dot concealer under your eyes, onto any spots and dab with your ring finger to blend it in. Don't wipe.

Crayon
Pick a thick crayon in a golden brown shade. It's subtle, suits everyone and is hard to get wrong. Draw the crayon across your upper lash line. Don't worry if it's a bit wobbly or seems too thick. The joy of a crayon is that it can be smudged and softened with your little finger or cotton bud, completely disguising any mistakes. Using the smudgy, slightly stained finger, trace the fingertip along the lower lash line to deposit a tiny amount of colour onto the skin.

Brows
Take any cheap clear mascara and use the wand to comb upwards, then downwards when you hit the natural arch.

Cheeks

Creme blush looks lovely on young skin and, if you choose one in a stick (like a big Bingo marker or Pritt Stick), a cinch to put on. Pink or apricot is ideal on all skin colours, berry is also lovely on Asian and black skins. For the most part, I'm not keen on shimmer – it will generally make you look as though you got your blush free on the cover of a magazine. Twist up the stick and dab the nib onto each cheek to make a circle of blush on each side. Use your middle finger to pat gently around the circle to blur the outline.

Lips

Use a tinted lip balm in roughly the same colour as your blusher. Apply it straight from the stick (you can also use this as your blusher if you're in a hurry or short of money, provided you don't suffer from acne, as they often contain shea butter or paraffin). If you prefer something more dressy, apply gloss, but again, it looks better if the shade vaguely matches your cheeks.

Lashes

Use a mascara in either brown or black. First wipe the wand on a tissue to avoid blobs. Looking down into a mirror, push the mascara wand upwards into your top lashes, wiggling it back and forth. Do not do that weird face lots of grown-up women do, where they open their mouth wide to put on mascara. It looks crazy and serves no purpose. Nip this utterly pointless habit in the bud now and you will thank me later (also, that hand wavy thing some women do when they start crying. Why? Make your generation break the cycle).

Glitter

Of course, glitter is not always appropriate but I also believe the opportunities to wear it are so scarce in later life that it seems a terrible waste not to occasionally embrace it now. While not suitable for school, dates or formal occasions (funerals: definite no), glitter is a fun thing to wear to parties and dances and makes any face seem dressed up. Be cautious, though; you're not a kid any more so lashings of sickly pink glitter looks really naff. Instead, pop some moisturiser or lip balm on your temples in a curved vertical line. Press on some glitter. Gold or silver looks especially lovely. Also nice is glittery crayon along the lashline, or glitter mascara stroked over black. Please note the ORs here. One area maximum – any more is not chic.

Teen beauty rules

Take it from someone who knows. You can go as crazy as you want, but make sure these things are locked down.

Have clean hair
If you have neither the time nor the inclination to do anything else with your appearance, make sure you have clean hair. Dirty hair always looks dirty, even if you think it doesn't, and it usually smells a bit gross too. It also doesn't help a spotty forehead. If you like the feel and styleability of day-old hair, then spray in some dry shampoo or mattifier after drying. Apparently Kate Moss lives by the Always Clean Hair rule – and she knows more about looking good than anyone.

Don't pluck your brows
The joy of experimenting with make-up is you can take it off again. Brows are not so flexible. Ask any group of grown women what they see as their biggest mistake and I guarantee one of them will say overplucking her eyebrows when young. Doing this can, and often does, result in a bald browline later on, or at least, sparse, thin brows that make you look a bit cross. What seems like a good option now will rob you of others later. You will bitterly regret going there. Please, please don't.

DON'T SHAVE YOUR BIKINI LINE

I hate to be a preaching mum, but I would really love it if no teenagers removed any hair from their bikini areas at all. Your pubic hair is new and it's natural and sort of brilliant. Let nature take its course and be proud of turning into a woman. Starting down the waxing path prompts a lifetime of hassle and takes your appearance back to girlhood at a time when things are starting to really get good. And don't ever let any boy (or girl) even express an opinion on what you should be doing with your genitals. They'd be bloody lucky to be seeing them in the first place. Wear your pubes with pride.

DON'T WEAR FOUNDATION

Even if you have acne, foundation is not the answer for young skin. Spots aside, your skin is currently looking better than it will ever look – plump, elastic, perky and full of life. Cover up blemishes with concealer, by all means, but don't mask your whole face in foundation. I promise you will one day look back at photographs and despair at your choice to wear base (I do). There's plenty of time to use it later when you might really need it.

DON'T BUY CELEBRITY PERFUMES

You may love Rihanna, Miley, Britney and co, but believe me when I say that most celebrities have little or no involvement in their perfumes until they're almost ready to go on sale. Most are sweet, sickly and synthetic-smelling, some are completely gross. Many are created by companies who have reduced you to a one-dimensional demographic of Lame Fangirl. There are hundreds, if not thousands, of lovely perfumes out there. Find one you love and confine your love of popstars to their records ('records' Hark at nana!), tickets and posters.

DON'T USE PORE STRIPS

You know those strips that you stick onto your blackheads then peel off, taking the disgusting bits with them? So satisfying, so gratifying, so pleasing. Unfortunately, I believe them to be very bad indeed. I believe they disrupt the delicate balance of your skin and cause more clogs, more blackheads, more spots, and leave them too clear and wide open, ready to catch more bacteria than they naturally would. Resist.

CLEANSE, CLEANSE, CLEANSE

Cleansing is the most important thing you can do for your skin, day to day. Please do it, even if you feel it's a drag. It will pay off. If you're too tired at night, then cleanse as soon as you get in from school, college or work so it's done. The important thing is that you do it twice a day and never sleep in your make-up. If you do, your skin will look worse. You'll get spots, blackheads and dryness. Get into the habit now and you'll feel extremely smug later on.

PROTECT YOUR SKIN

Sunscreen probably feels like decades away, especially if you like to be brown, but most sun damage occurs before your 21st birthday. Using a high-protection sunscreen (any that protects against both UVA and UVB is fine) will really help premature skin ageing in the future. It may well feel like starting a pension before you've ever started work, but the benefits of SPF will show themselves sooner than you think. If I could change one thing in life, I would not spend my best friend Rachel's sweet sixteenth on a beach in Port Einon, wearing a really crap bra and factor zero oil. I can still see now where I burnt my face. Learn from my abject stupidity.

DON'T GO ON A SUNBED

No, no, no, no. Sunbeds inflict TWELVE times the level of UVA (the skin-ageing rays) on your poor skin. I'm horrified they even still exist, before I even dare think about the fact that they're suddenly so popular with young women. They are not good for you, whether you are super pale or mega dark. If you must tan, get it from a tube.

BE KIND TO YOUR SKIN

Your skin is your body's largest organ and certainly the most attractive. Value it and show it some respect. Don't scrub it like a tin bath, thinking punishment will cause it to submit. Don't starve it of moisture because it's misbehaving, and don't roast it like a turkey because you think it's too pale. And please, please don't start smoking. You will absolutely rue the day you invited it to the party, only to see it trash the joint.

DON'T GET A TATTOO

I adore tattoos (I have two) but thank God I didn't get one until I a) could afford a really great artist, b) had frankly nothing more exciting to do with my time than research my design, artist, placement and theme thoroughly, and c) had come to realise that few teen passions – from romantic partners and best friends to favourite bands and holiday resorts – last as long as a tattoo. Tattoos can be wonderful – I am very much pro any form of creative self-expression – but now is not the time. I promise you'll be glad you waited.

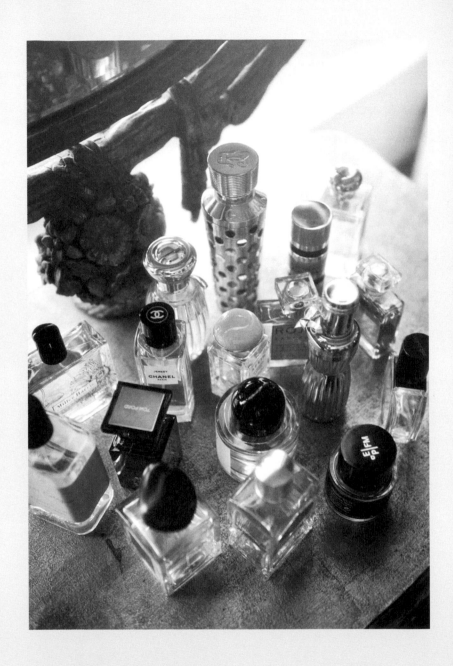

PERFUME

'A woman's perfume tells more about
her than her handwriting.'
Christian Dior

My first memory of perfume is the day I decided to make my own. I took my mother's black glass bottle of Biba cologne (cheap then, now worth fortunes) and poured it into the toilet of her little flat. I poured apple shampoo on top of it, then some TCP and my stepfather's Paco Rabanne, and was stirring it all together with an upside-down toilet brush when my mother walked into the tiny bathroom. It was my first foray into perfumery and I've no idea how I was permitted to live to tell the tale.

Perfume is my favourite beauty product and has been since a few years after my home perfumery experiment, when I was around ten years old. I was sitting upstairs reading when my mother returned home slightly tipsy from a wine-tasting in France (I suspect her condition was instrumental here), and handed me a little white cotton-paper bag containing a box, perfectly giftwrapped in thick black and white houndstooth paper and a white bow. In it was a bottle of Miss Dior – my first perfume. I became instantly and enduringly hooked.

You'll find most perfume enthusiasts have memories such as these, formative experiences that kickstarted a lifelong obsession with scent. This isn't surprising when you consider that smell is the most evocative of all the senses. One whiff can transport us back to our first classroom, to our grandmother's ironing pile, to a childhood holiday and our first proper snog. Scent actually makes us feel things – comforted, relaxed, moved, tearful, happy – just as paintings, books and music do. Perfume also allows me to choose who I am today, much in the same way as a red lipstick does, or dark eyes, or a severe pony tail or sexy bed hair. But unlike any other beauty product, scent is a vocal companion. I can choose not to look in a mirror, or to quickly change my lipstick shade, but one has to hang out with a perfume throughout the day. It's important to love the one you're with, so to speak.

Spraying scent is not like cleaning my teeth – an unconscious reflex or muscle memory. It's a deliberate decision based on how I feel, what I'm wearing, who I'm seeing and how I want them to react to me. If I want to feel sexy, I might wear Frederic Malle's Carnal Flower. If I wish to communicate elegance and refinement, I might choose Guerlain Mitsouko. If I want to feel kickass and go-getting, I'll wear YSL Rive

Gauche, if I'm down and want to be reminded that all will ultimately be well, I spray on Malle's L'eau d'Hiver and inhale deeply. If I meet friends for a casual lunch, on goes Miller Harris' Le Petit Grain with some mascara and lip balm. If I go for dinner, I might wear the unobtrusive but dressy Rive d'Ambre by Tom Ford with killer make-up and a little black dress. And in any situation, from the unexpected to the familiar, there's always Chanel No5 – the olfactory equivalent of backbone, a strict and impossibly glamorous aunt who remains calm and wholly appropriate in a crisis, whatever the complexity behind her eyes. To me, wearing No5 is like carrying a loaded pistol in my knickers. I am always prepared.

I feel sad when so many people tell me they don't like perfume and I'm afraid I become like some nana who believes the parish bachelor who still lives with his mother at 50 and arranges the church flowers on weekends 'just hasn't met the right girl yet'. I also think that my generation spawned a great number of perfume haters because our mothers wore 1980s power scents that caused instant migraines in innocent bystanders. Poison, Paris, Passion, Ysatis, LouLou, Eden and my worst, the inimitable Giorgio Beverly Hills (which my mother once spilled in her Mini, instantly rendering me transportless for the remainder of my teens, so intolerable and nauseating was the smell) – all were sprayed liberally and inconsiderately for the best part of a decade, permanently damaging many people's goodwill towards perfume. This should be overcome. It is simply not possible that you don't like nice fragrances, unless you have no sense of smell. There is a perfume for you out there and with every day you don't look for it, time's a-wasting.

So how to start your own fragrance wardrobe? We've all fallen for a beautiful ad campaign, a gorgeous bottle or magazine write-up, and to a certain degree, all of those things can contribute to the magic of perfumery. But it's essential to try to ignore them in choosing a perfume, not least because only perfumers with the money for the fanfare can join in, while many brilliant fragrances on a tighter budget are consequently ignored.

But for a consumer, at least, scent is the most egalitarian product. You don't have to be beautiful, young or thin to smell a million dollars.

Every woman can enjoy perfume – she may just need help finding the right one in a sea of fancy ad campaigns, and probably about 50 quid in her purse. With this, patience and curiosity, she can find the perfect fragrance. A scent that is personal, elegant and, crucially (at least to me), one that can't be identified from a hundred paces. The array of perfumes available can be quite dizzying, so here's how to get started.

How to choose a perfume

I generally have a great deal of respect for beauty counter staff but I'm afraid the buying of perfume is the one time I'd advise you to ignore anything they say. The average sales consultant is trained to sell perfume in the same way she sells nail polish – as a lucrative add-on to up the unit sales. A great make-up artist she may well be, but it's unlikely she really knows her scent beyond the training notes and ingredient lists she's been given. Where you will find staff with knowledge and love for perfume is in a specialist perfumery. I understand why this causes some anxiety in those who've never before shopped for perfume beyond the duty-free supermarket, but really, the staff in shops like Les Senteurs, Roja Dove Haute Parfumerie, Miller Harris, Ormonde Jayne, Liberty perfumery and L'Artisan Parfumeur are, in my experience, incredibly kind and welcoming – almost to the point of being delighted that you're showing an interest in their passion. Because these people understand perfume, they know you cannot be expected to make a decision on the spot, they appreciate that samples are important, that some guidance may be useful. They tend to be unpushy and play the long game. Do go in on a quiet weekday and either browse independently or let them take you in hand. Tell them which smells you normally like, whether it's another perfume, your favourite flower, herb or food. They will make suggestions based on your answers and take you through a trialling process, tinkering here and there – less sweet but just as fruity, a little more leathery, less wood and more spice – until you arrive at The One. You will learn a lot. I promise you it will be a worthwhile experience.

In any case – whether you're shopping in an airport lounge,

department store or specialist boutique, staff can only do so much. This is your perfume and must be to your nose's liking. There is no substitute for smelling and there's only so much that can be accomplished in a day. I find that after eight perfumes, my nose becomes wholly confused and shuts up shop. Any further testing is a waste of time, so I try to be discerning from the off. I am attracted to a scent I haven't tested via a number of different routes. Often I've been intrigued by online reviews on forums like fragrantica.com or MakeupAlley.com, sometimes I will write about perfume I love and a reader will suggest another I haven't tried. Sometimes I've heard friends or colleagues mention a perfume in either an effusive or disparaging way and want to form my own opinion. Very often it's the name of a perfume, which seems shallow and irrelevant, but with little else to go on (bottle is certainly no indicator and nor are ingredients really – there are chocolate and almond cakes that are light, moist, springy and rich, and there are chocolate and almond cakes that taste like twice-washed cardboard dipped in cocoa dust), words appeal at least to my curiosity. Whether they wilfully give nothing away (Molecule 01 and Chanel No22, for example) or are wholly literal in their approach (Malle's Lipstick Rose, Prada's Infusion D'Iris, Jo Malone's English Pear & Freesia), a name gives me something to go on before I lean in for a sniff.

Before you go shopping, pour a little freshly ground coffee into a ziplock bag and put it in your handbag. To test a perfume, I always in the first instance use perfume strips. Any good department store or perfumery will have plenty of these from which you can help yourself. These are made from absorbent 'blotting'-type paper that give as true an impression of a scent as possible without smelling it on your skin. Use a pencil or biro to write the perfume name on the strip so you don't forget later, then spray on both sides. Wave the strip to help lose the hit of alcohol, then sniff. The smell will change dramatically over the next 15–20 minutes, so don't be rash, but a good first impression is encouraging. Before you move on to the next, open the ziplock of coffee and inhale. The aroma will clear your head and act as a nasal cleanser to avoid confusing subsequent perfumes. You can keep doing this until everything starts to smell the same, then stop for lunch. Revisit the by-now matured strip samples and pick out a couple you especially like. You'll notice that the odd strip may have already lost its smell almost altogether. This is a bad sign and a sure indicator that it will do the same on your wrist and need to be reapplied hourly. Who can be bothered? Eliminate it. Some samples may have become extremely sweet and somewhat headache-inducing. Bin them. Others, if you're lucky, will have softened, enriched, perhaps become more powdery, with different elements becoming more prominent than originally apparent. All this is a good sign. If you like what you smell, it's worth allowing these through to the finals and onto your skin.

As with buying art or antiques, the secret to buying fragrance is in buying what you instinctively love and not to get too bogged down in what you feel you should like. There's a mood for everything and you could be missing out in categorising yourself too decisively. For example, I think unfussy and elegant clothes with a little unexpected detail or two lends itself to something like Frederic Malle's L'eau d'Hiver, which I absolutely adore, but sometimes I want to put on a leopard-print dress and feel a bit whorish. Suddenly the creamy, soft and ambrosial smell of almond milk isn't going to cut it and I want some big, blousey Oriental scent no man would dare buy his mother. When I want to land a new job, or take back a defective toaster, the quiet chic of figgy Diptyque Philosykos is not going to adequately fight my corner. Meanwhile, I have broadly expensive tastes, but I love Coty L'Aimant (under a tenner) and am aroused by the smell of Old Spice. It's important to keep an open mind like this because the only people who really want to pigeonhole you are the perfume companies. People, mercifully, are more complex than that.

Finding your formula

Many people don't know the difference between eau de toilette and perfume, beyond the difference in price. Here's a brief guide to each.

Pure perfume oil

Single-note oils like those bought in health-food shops and aromatherapist suppliers aren't perfumes, they're just oils that happen to smell nice. A pure 100 per cent perfume oil made by a perfumer is rare and would almost certainly smell foul or, at least, not anything like itself. A pure perfume is a bit like trying to read a document in a zip file. The alcohol and water helps it to decompress and expand into something coherent and readable.

Perfume or parfum

People will often describe perfume as 'stronger' and while I know what they mean, it's misleading. What perfume, parfum or 'extrait' is is the most concentrated juice, containing a higher percentage (between 25 and 40 per cent) of perfume oils and aromatic ingredients (the 'compound'). Perfume contains less alcohol than its dilutes – eau de parfum and eau de toilette. But none of this necessarily means a 'stronger' smell, more a richer and longer-lasting one. Often, a perfume actually smells softer than its dilutes. A connoisseur will generally prefer a perfume formulation, seeing as how it's probably closest to a perfumer's original vision, but I think in all honesty, I broadly prefer…

Eau de parfum

EDP has around 15–20 per cent concentration of aromatic compound. It seems to me to be a happy medium. It doesn't stain clothes as badly (I once had a terrible mishap with some Guerlain perfume and a borrowed silk dress) but still lasts long enough to soften and develop well before it needs a top-up. Its less terrifying cost means I can spray it on with some abandon without feeling like Imelda Marcos, and I know that if I'm wearing it publicly, I'm not unduly forcing my scent onto others.

EAU DE TOILETTE

A perfume concentration of about 10 per cent, EDT is substantially cheaper than perfume but will need to be resprayed at least twice a day to keep it alive, making it a dubious economy. EDT always smells a little sharper to me – it comes on strong, but fails to hang around for cuddles afterwards. Like any fleeting encounter, it's often better than nothing but is no substitute for something more substantial.

EAU DE COLOGNE

Here's where I am inconsistent. While I'm not a fan of EDT, I adore cologne, absolutely love it. It's an even lighter (typically around 5 per cent concentration), citrus and crisp fragrance type which, though born in Germany, smells very French to me. Unlike the other dilutions, cologne rarely has a parent perfume and operates more as a scent unto itself. It's a fresh, fleeting and alcoholic formula that's hugely uplifting. It's like a party guest who runs in, tells some great jokes, makes a toast and swiftly leaves before even taking off its coat. It's extremely uplifting stuff, unpretentious and familiar. It's also very sexy on both men and women and is a real tonic during sticky summers. I've no time for people who sneer at cologne. They are missing out badly.

SOLID PERFUMES

Hmmm. My experience of these pretty, handbag-friendly compacts of perfume has been very mixed. You might expect a solid wax of perfume oil to be highly concentrated and long lasting, but this has only sometimes been my experience – many seem enveloped in beeswax, paraffin or some such thing. Others are very lovely, but what is true across the board is that these leave greasy stains on fine fabrics and attract lint from knitwear. It's not chic so it's a no from me.

Some cheap and unexpected smells i adore

Everyday products with the most wonderful fragrance

Pantene shampoo and conditioner

....

Original Nivea Creme

....

Yardley English Lavender

....

Badedas bath foam

....

Cheap apple shampoo like Alberto Balsam or supermarket own brand

....

Retro soaps like Imperial Leather, Camay or Pear's

....

Max Factor Crème Puff face powder

....

Huge tubs of cheap hair gel

....

Carmex lip balm

....

Hawaiian Tropic suntan oil

....

Johnson & Johnson's Baby Lotion

....

Elnett Hairspray

....

Pond's Cold Cream

....

Deep Heat injury spray

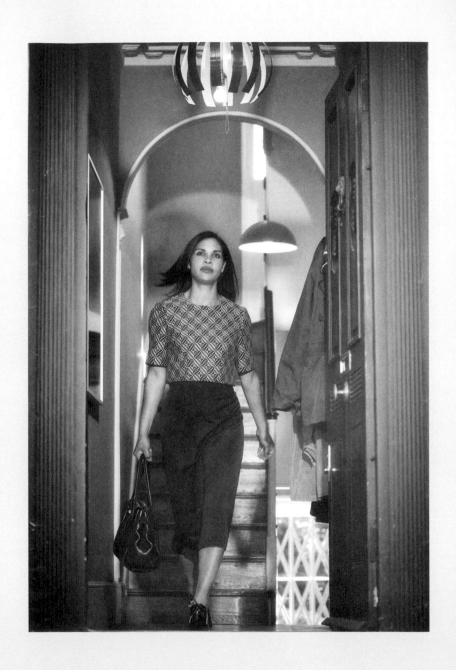

BEAUTY AND THE CAREERWOMAN

'I think dress, hairstyle and make-up are the crucial
factors in projecting an attractive persona and give one
the chance to enhance one's best physical features.'
Vivienne Westwood

My work make-up is completely different to the face I present when I'm at home. For me, work make-up is a bit like perfume and high heels – not essential, but they help me feel businesslike and able to put my best foot forward (my partner would never attend a meeting unshaven, I imagine this is much the same impulse). Make-up also provides a sort of demarcation; I know that when my pyjamas are off, lipstick is on and my hair looks half decent, the day has begun and it really is time to stop dicking about on the internet and earn some money. If you feel just as confident going into the workplace bare-faced, then by all means do that, but I suppose I use my appearance to demonstrate that I have an eye for detail, am always prepared to make an effort and that I understand the importance of first impressions.

There are other ways by which you can do this, of course, but if I can indulge my passion and also feel good as part of the bargain, then why not do so through my appearance? It's just another tool that I'm lucky enough to have at my disposal. Some people play squash with their colleagues to get ahead (I'd rather die), others go to the pub (I've got kids and my own friends I already don't see enough). But clothes, hair and make-up, I can do.

All that said, if people see your make-up before your work, then you have a big problem. Your appearance is not what you're being paid for (unless you're a model, of course) and presenting yourself smartly and appropriately should act merely as a frame to the main attraction – your talent and skills. This can be tricky to get right. With the emphasis within office environments becoming more and more creative, along with dress-down Fridays and ambiguous dress codes, women have been left confused about what constitutes appropriate professional make-up. When to go bold? When to lay off? Which looks scream power and success and which represent the beauty equivalent of a bikini and stripper heels?

For a basic work face, I recommend the look described in the chapter on Public Displays of Grooming. It's solid, smart and appropriate to most workplaces, and it is also pretty versatile – you can switch the shade of eye crayon according to your outfit, swap the tinted moisturiser for foundation if you need to look immaculate all day, and so on. There will also be times when you'll want to ramp things up a bit for added impact (asking for a pay rise, laying down the law, making a big presentation). For these occasions, I'd suggest one of the following, but never both simultaneously:

Power lips
Full base of foundation, concealer and powder. A simple chocolate-brown eyeliner pencil, black mascara and groomed brows, pale pink or rose powder blusher. Lips lined sharply with red or Bordeaux pencil and filled in with non-shimmery matching lipstick, blotted, reapplied, then blotted. Red nails are optional but effective, especially if you are giving a presentation (the audience's natural eyeline will follow your hands as you talk).

Strong eyes
Irrespective of skin colour, choose three eyeshadows in ivory, taupe and chocolate brown. One should have a very slight shimmer for blending ease. Brush the ivory over the entire lid, from lashline to brow. Using a crease brush (MAC's 219 is the best ever), stroke the taupe in an arc a fraction above the crease. Pivot your hand like a windscreen wiper or compass for the perfect shape. Use a liner brush to apply the chocolate-brown shadow along the lash line, top and bottom. Smudge and soften the lines with the crease brush. Add mascara. Wear with a nude lipstick with a slight sheen and a matching blusher (creme or powder).

Deskside essentials

Keep these beauty staples in your pedestal cabinet for post-lunch and between-meetings touch-ups.

Powder compact
Essential for keeping shine at bay on all skin types, and a lifesaver for menopausal women who often find skin becomes sweaty and greasy-looking after an hour or so. Lightly coat a velour puff with powder and gently dab – don't wipe – your nose, chin and forehead.

Dry shampoo
A mini can of this is just the thing if your hair has become flat or stringy, or if you want to give it some extra height and bulk for meetings in which you want to appear really formidable. Spray it into your roots, leave for a few moments, then massage into your roots like a normal shampoo. Brush it out, then style as you wish.

Lipstick
It is far, far better to wear no lipstick than one that has smudged, faded, bled or clung to the rim of your lips, avoiding the middle like some wallflower at a school dance. Personally, I would never attend a meeting without it and so touch-ups throughout the day are essential. Nude (lighter on white skin, richer on dark) and rose shades are great generic work looks on all skin tones, though I would always keep a red handy for when you need to show colleagues you mean business.

MINTS

Bad breath in the workplace = end of days. Don't allow yourself to be distracted by paranoia. Pop a mint before meetings or whenever you're working in very close proximity to a colleague. Be free and easy about offering them around too. It's the international code for 'please address your oxygen output' and far better than leaving someone to feel dreadful when they become aware of their halitosis later on.

DIPPY NAIL POLISH REMOVER POT

Genius invention for removing chipped polish on the move, without any need for cotton wool. Simply dip your fingers into the hole for a couple of seconds then pull them out clean (I would still do this in the Ladies – the dippy pots smell the same as classic remover and may not go down well with colleagues). This should always be done when nail polish is past its best. Clean nails are perfectly acceptable, chipped ones make you look sloppy and inattentive to detail.

EMERY BOARD

Jagged nails ruin tights, thus ruining your day (or life, if they're Wolfords). Always have an emery board handy.

MINI HAIRSPRAY

For fixing styles into place, preventing hair static and spraying onto tights on days when your frock clings to them.

Cotton buds and small bottle of micellar lotion

A lunch-hour downpour can cover your face in mascara, too much coffee can smudge your lips. Cotton buds and micellar will sort any mishap in seconds without ruining any surrounding make-up. You can also use the buds to apply eyeshadow if you're going out after work.

Hairbrush

If you don't carry a hairbrush in your bag, you'll need to leave one at work. A quick lunchtime brush has an instantly uplifting effect. It makes me feel neat, smart, more awake and ready to go back to work.

Antibac hand gel and hand cream

I'm not a hygiene freak but even I find most offices a bit gross in places. An antibacterial gel helps. Always use the hand cream afterwards, as the gels can be drying.

Perfume

I always have a scent in my bag but if you don't carry one with you, keep one somewhere handy at work. Nothing focuses the mind for presentations, meetings and other front-facing stuff like a great perfume. Keep it polite, though – no one wants a face full of strong, heady pong. An eau de parfum of something unobtrusive is best – save the full-on sexy scents for nighttime.

WORKPLACE NO-NOS

Different workplace environments mean exceptions to every rule. Nurses and doctors are often not permitted to wear nail polish or their hair down, barristers rarely attend court without full make-up, while fashion-industry workers know that absolutely anything goes provided it's on-brand. But very generally speaking, the following looks represent professional beauty faux pas.

NAIL ART

Unless you work in a nail salon or fashion environment, nail art is distracting, fussy and too girly for professional wear. It's also completely unacceptable in food preparation and service jobs. No one wants to find a rogue pink crystal or Mickey Mouse decal floating in their macchiato.

EXCESSIVE SHIMMER

Okay, as a basic rule, I believe anything that makes you look young and inexperienced is not a great image in the workplace, nor is anything that looks as though it was hauled straight into work from a nightclub. Shimmery make-up is distracting, girlie and inappropriate for day.

JAMMY LIP GLOSS

Wear tinted balm, a satiny gloss or proper lipstick. Something sticky and pouty is naff, young and high maintenance. It also makes workwear look a bit cheap. You're not at the beach or disco.

FALSE EYELASHES

Unless you've undergone chemo, false lashes in the workplace seem try-hard and to some may suggest your priorities are somewhat out of whack. If lashes are your thing, wear a false-effect mascara and apply two coats, or consider semi-permanent extensions.

WET HAIR

Men and women who do this might as well wear a sandwich board saying 'I REALLY CAN'T BE BOTHERED'. Ensuring your hair is dry after showering isn't vanity, it's basic grooming. To not bother looks sloppy and lazy. Invest in a microfibre towel to wrap your wet hair in – they're so absorbent that your hair will be almost dry by the time you've eaten your cereal. When you get to work, nip to the Ladies and tip your head upside down underneath the hand dryer. If you really have no time to dry your hair then don't wash it that morning, instead use a dry shampoo or consider washing it the night before.

ANTI-SOCIAL PERFUME

Be considerate to your co-workers and avoid pungent, heady scents that alter the taste of any coffee consumed within 30 feet of you. Perfumes like Angel, Poison, Giorgio Beverly Hills, LouLou, Opium and Samsara are not okay for work. Choose something soft, elegant and light and spray sparingly – remember, it's normal for you to lose the ability to smell your own perfume after long-term use. Ask a trusted friend if you're not sure.

Dress-down Fridays

Ugh. An American import that seems reluctant to go away. It seems to me that if a more casual look is fine in your working environment on one day a week, then it should be perfectly acceptable on the other four too. I can see it makes sense that when you are wearing more casual clothes your make-up can be toned down too, but I would still always keep a decent lipstick about my person. Even if the rest of your face is very subtly made-up, a lipstick immediately scales things up when you need it. You will never feel underdressed in a bold lipstick, even if you are wearing jeans and a T-shirt, and you will always feel noticed.

Interview make-up

Interview make-up, if worn, should be smart, grown-up and well applied. Hair should be freshly washed and blow-dried, nails must be spotlessly clean and either left bare or painted with a clear or subtle polish (rose works well). Now is not the time to be bold and be outshone by your make-up, so avoid red lips, black liner, fancy nails and coloured eyeshadow. Instead, choose nudes – and by that I mean shades that are naturally present in any skin shade, from pale ivory to rose pink, to medium apricot to darkest espresso brown. All of these work on every skin tone – you really can't go wrong within that palette. If you're useless at applying eyeshadow, skip it and use a crayon. If you can't put on lipstick neatly, use a tinted balm. Badly applied make-up is the physical equivalent of blagging on your CV; it's much better to do what you can well than pretend to have skills you don't. It'll just look sloppy.

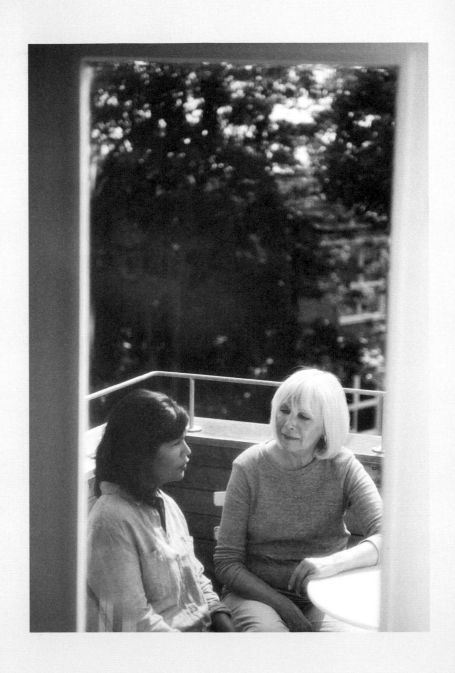

MATURE BEAUTY

'Beautiful young people are accidents of nature,
but beautiful old people are works of art.'
Eleanor Roosevelt

I can barely type the words 'age appropriate' without my blood pressure shifting sharply up a notch. The term, bandied about by people who consider themselves too polite and right-on to say 'Mutton dressed as lamb', is just another way of asking women over 45 to know their place and to go and be quiet, bland and sexless over there, while the young women get to briefly enjoy their superior appearances.

Being over 45 does not mean no longer having fun with make-up, nor does it mean retiring into a sort of demure silver-fox cliché from a denture-glue commercial. You still have every right to look fabulous, sexy and like you, you just may now have more obstacles to navigate on the way. Eyeliner, once standing tall in sharp flicks, can now jump into the eye crease in a wobbly smudge, lipstick that once sat neatly on your mouth can now migrate through fine lines and make it look a bit cat's bottom. Skin can lose its perky colour, moisture, even tone and firmness, menopause can force make-up to slide off the face. This is all normal, annoying, but manageable with the right products and techniques. It's not about swapping your identity, but about enjoying what you've always had in a way that's flattering to what you have now.

An older woman who still delights in beauty makes me happier than anything. Ninety-two-year-old Baroness Trumpington, with her desk full of bright Rimmel nail polishes, Lauren Bacall with her thick arched brows, Debbie Harry and Brix Smith-Start with their resolutely white-blonde bobs and bold lips all represent to me a far more enjoyable way of growing older than in some generic hairdo, frightened lipstick and sensible shoes from the back of the Sunday supplement (as artist Sue Kreitzman put so eloquently, 'Beige is the colour of death. Don't wear beige. It might kill you'). They remain themselves and in possession of their signature style and spirit. That's what makes them beautiful and what conveniently cannot be obscured by a few wrinkles. They don't look like young women; they look like beautiful mature ones. That is the key.

Of course, it's all very well telling women to enjoy their identities, but during menopause and beyond it can seem as though society has changed yours without prior consultation. Clients and readers tell me they suddenly feel invisible, unattractive, unfeminine and unsure of how they should look. This is often where advice and clear instruction is useful. Did you know that a sparkly crayon is your new best friend, or that teeth whitening will knock off more years than a jawlift? Or that a big arse equals a relatively line-free face? Or that lying upwards about your age is far more sensible than lying downwards? Or that what I call a reverse lip liner will stop your lipstick going Dot Cotton? I will take you through what needs to change, what should stay and what never to waste your precious money on.

Mature Beauty: The Rules

Bin the magnifying mirror

Of all the women I see over 40 years old, I'd say 90 per cent of them complain of enlarged pores. Of that number, fewer than 5 per cent actually have anything to worry about. Pores do become bigger as we get older – you're not imagining it – but what is crucial for all of us to remember is that no one, literally no one, views our faces in the same way we do. We scrutinise in a magnifying mirror, noticing every last pore. Meanwhile even our closest friends merely glance in our direction, appreciate briefly the whole picture of our appearance, then get on with their own business. They'd be no more likely to notice an enlarged pore than a speck of dust on a cardi.

It's really important that you don't fall down the rabbit hole of self-scrutiny in your mature years because, truly, you will be fighting a losing battle. Each month, your face will show new evidence of the ageing process, much of it uncontrollable, and you will drive yourself crackers, like someone holding their hand over the leak in a colander. That way madness lies.

Don't get too thin

Pick a weight and try to stay roughly there, give or take a few puddings. Drastic weight loss or a very low body mass index is ageing to the face, makes skin sag more easily and develop lines more quickly. A healthy amount of fat is very useful as scaffolding under the skin and gives the impression of greater fullness, plumping out lines and creases. To paraphrase Barbara Cartland, old-age beauty really is often a case of choosing between face and arse. I'd choose face on the grounds that I never want anyone to see me from behind and think I'm 30, only to realise I'm ancient when I turn around. Much more satisfying to have a vibrant face.

Brighten grey

There's nothing wrong with grey hair (nor with dyeing it), but the loss of hair pigment can drain the face of colour. Brightening the grey with silver really helps perk up your skin tone. Use blue or lavender-toned shampoo to remove brassiness and dullness (Aveda Blue Malva and A Touch of Silver are both great) and consider the possibility of dyeing it completely silver – it avoids the whole in-betweeny salt-and-pepper phase that makes you look older than 100 per cent grey does. Don't be convinced that grey hair must be short, that is nonsense – long, silvery hair can look striking and feminine.

Exercise

Wherever you're at on the scales, it is extremely beneficial to your appearance to exercise. People who move around more just look better. A good exercise regime will also keep muscles firm and where they should be, holding up your face, and aids circulation, improving dullness and grey skin. Weight training, boxing, running, brisk walking (especially outside), sex and swimming are all great for your health and, consequently, your appearance. I understand completely why exercise seems boring, but just walking short journeys instead of taking the car can make a huge difference quite quickly. Things like yoga and pilates are wonderful for helping to keep the joints working fluidly.

REMOVE FACIAL HAIR

A friend of mine visited her dying great-grandmother every day in hospital, purely in order to pluck the chin hairs she knew her great-gran loathed. I find it very moving the way women understand this stuff and know it to be meaningful. I really hope that when my time comes, someone will visit my bedside brandishing tweezers and possibly a hipflask. In the meantime, I will most certainly be doing it myself. Noticeable facial hair is ageing and given that most women don't want it when young, to start leaving it there can look as though one has given up. For upper lip, threading is my preferred method (see Brows) but cream is painless and can be used at home. IPL is a lasting solution and may well be worth it for persistent hair growth, though the technology won't work on white or grey hairs. Chin hairs are uniquely fast-sprouting as we get older. Sometimes the only way to keep up is via plucking. Buy good tweezers (Rubis or Tweezerman) to make light of the job.

MOISTURISE

The best way to make your skin soft, supple and glowing is via a moisturiser suited to your skin type, applied twice a day. I personally feel the most reliable mature skin creams are by mega brands bought in supermarkets – Olay, Nivea, L'Oréal Paris and so on – since they seem to take normal older women most seriously, not to mention the fact they have almost unlimited funds to throw at research and development. They often contain proven ingredients like retinol and hyaluronic acid and more speculative technology like antioxidants, all for a not-too-horrific price. Massage in generously in relatively firm upward strokes. Finish by pinching your cheeks to add a little flush. In the evenings I would add a facial oil (rosehip is marvellous on skin over 45 and can be bought in health- food shops and chemists). Massage in well, don't be puny about it. It's also worth treating yourself to regular facial massage – I do believe they help. Look to YouTube for some good tutorials, and consider buying a massage roller – a small painter-style tool with textured wheels to give consistent, even pressure.

TAKE CARE OF YOUR TEETH

People are wrong in thinking wrinkles cause a woman to look old (see Anti-ageing for specific advice on these). Wrinkles are fine, they can be nice and are wholly copeable-with for most women. What ages your appearance is crap teeth and hair. When both look healthy and vibrant, so do you. There is nothing more ageing than poor teeth. A brownish, decaying mouth can put ten years on you. Visit your dentist regularly and if you are to invest some cash in improving your appearance, spend it here. See a hygienist every 12 weeks for a proper clean and consider whitening once every two years. I have often told women on the verge of a facelift to divert the cash towards their teeth. It's a far wiser, safer and more convincing investment.

THINK ABOUT REMOVING THREAD VEINS

Red veins around your nose and eyes are extremely common in older age. They are harmless and can to a large degree be covered by an opaque concealer (see Foundation on how to cover anything), but when on show, they can age your face unnecessarily. Fortunately, they're pretty easy to remove. For about the same price as a haircut and a full head of highlights, a thread vein can be removed permanently at a skin clinic. Ask your GP for a recommendation.

LOOK AFTER YOUR FEET

Feet show age faster than everywhere else, but fortunately this is one of the areas of the body that is most responsive to a little care. Get a foot file and file down hard skin regularly (about once a week). It's painless and makes a remarkable difference. Rinse after filing, slather on very rich foot cream (heel balm if the skin is really hard), then put on some cotton socks for bed. It is also a good investment to visit a chiropodist a couple of times a year. I never enter the summer months without first getting a medi-pedi – having someone take to your feet with a scalpel is, shamefully, better than sex.

LIE UPWARDS ABOUT YOUR AGE

I will never understand why so many women of 60 plus seem so set on the world thinking they are, in fact, a girl of only 40. Why lie downwards? It's mad and only makes people immediately wonder where the hell life went so badly wrong. If you must lie about it, it is much more impressive and fabulous to say you're five years older then have people gasp in admiration at how young and vibrant you look for your (fake) age. 'Seventy? Good grief, you barely look sixty! How marvellous, what's your secret?', etc. They'll be so impressed they'll never notice you fudging over historical detail.

THINGS TO AVOID AFTER FORTY-FIVE

Wear what you want, but know these things aren't helping.

SHIMMER EYESHADOW

There's no doubt that shimmery shadow makes crepey eyelids look much more so. It also accentuates dryness. But I would advise caution in switching to matte full time because it can look a little dull on the face when it's already lost some light. Instead, try lining matte-shadowed eyes with a shimmery crayon or pencil. The liner will add some shine, sparkle and light without any shimmer settling on the lids and highlighting wrinkles. Bobbi Brown, Charlotte Tilbury, Barry M, Topshop, Smashbox, Clinique and Laura Mercier all make good ones.

BLACK EYELINER

If black eyeliner is your thing and you can't imagine life without it, then you carry on. It will always be a good look, whether it's Anita Pallenberg's groupie smudges or Dame Margot Fonteyn's ballerina liquid flicks. But if you feel your eyes are starting to look sunken and lined, the fastest fix may be to swap your black liner for chocolate brown, emerald green, khaki, amethyst, navy or bronze. You'll still get the darkness and definition, but the look will be softer, more flattering and more youthful. Avoid lining inside, i.e. in the waterline, too. And always smudge your lower line with a clean brush, cotton bud or pinky finger to avoid any hard edges.

CUTTING OFF YOUR HAIR

I've no idea who first decreed that all women over 35 should cut off their hair, but I'd be mustard-keen to knock them out. Apart from being patronising, reductive and offensive (the unspoken rule seems to be that mature women should take up as little space as possible and reject their former identities in favour of making jam that's free of rogue hairs), it's just plain wrong. If short hair suits you and how you live, great, but if you look best with longer hair, it can look very youthful and feminine. Keep it. The last thing women need is to return to the days when all women over 50 sported the same short, white cauliflower crown 'do. The condition of your long hair may become coarser, though, so treat it to regular moisturising treatments.

SHIMMERY NAIL POLISH

Frosty nails make hands look older and dryer. Choose a creamy finish without shimmer – if you want to add sparkle you can safely do so with a glittery top coat. Also, anything blue-based (blue-reds, cool purples, pastel blues, cerise pink, etc.) will pick up the blue and green in visible veins on your hands and accentuate them. Corals, orangey reds, taupe, chocolate brown, warm wines and soft pinks all work better.

HAIR-GROWTH SUPPLEMENTS

I don't believe in them, quite simply. If they worked then men the world over would pop them like Tic Tacs. Hair thinning and loss happen to most of us as we age, so make the best of things by asking your hairdresser to add in multi-tonal highlights, which act as an optical illusion of thickness. Always use a volumising shampoo and a light conditioner (I swear by Elvive and Swell on my thin hair), and blow dry using some mousse or volumising spray first. Invest in a rotating barrel brush too – Babyliss make the best ones.

THINGS THAT WORK ESPECIALLY WELL ON MATURE FACES

Anyone can use these, but they come into their own on older women.

PORE BALMS

These are temporary fillers, plugging pores with harmless silicone and creating a smoother base for make-up. After skincare, you dab them on with your middle finger and pat, don't wipe, or the balm may disintegrate. Then smooth on foundation. Clinique, Sensai, Dior, Benefit, L'Oréal Paris and Clarins make good ones.

A HAND CREAM WITH SUNSCREEN

People often protect their faces from sun damage while completely ignoring their hands, but applying sunscreen is very wise if you would like to avoid age spots. If you have existing spots, they will usually become much darker in hot weather, so slather on plenty of sunscreen before going out. At night, use a handcream that contains proven anti-ageing ingredients like retinol, to treat any damage that has already been done.

LIP PLUMPERS

These plump lips and fill in fine lines simultaneously and can work rather well, albeit temporarily. Some tingle when first applied, which can be annoying, but they don't cause any harm so it's worth waiting for the sensation to pass. Apply after base make-up and leave a few minutes before applying lipstick. I love Guerlain's because it doesn't tingle, but Molton Brown and Laura Mercier's are also good.

EYESHADOW PRIMERS

I am devoted to these. You know when your eyeliner transfers onto your eyelids? This is a common problem as we get older and eyelids begin to hood and can be helped enormously by a shadow primer. After your base but before eye make-up, tap a small amount of eye primer over the entire lid. Leave to set for a few moments before applying shadow. The best eye primers are by Urban Decay, Smashbox, Tom Ford, Stila, Clinique and Bare Minerals. Avoid coloured ones; what you need is a translucent, matte, universal shade that disappears on the skin.

LIP LINERS

People are snotty about lip liner. This is a huge mistake. Liner helps stop lipstick bleed and defines a blurring natural lip line (both common in mature women). Your pencil should always match your lipstick (that dark line/pale lip look of yore makes everyone look horrific) but if you can't find a match, opt for an invisible wax one. Body Shop, Estée Lauder, MAC, Cargo, Lipstick Queen and pro beauty supply stores (see Specialist Shops) all sell them. Trace the pencil around your natural lip line then fill in with lipstick.

PRIMER

Primers are great on older skins as they fix a number of common problems. They form a grippy base for make-up to stop it migrating during a hot flash, they smooth any unevenness on the surface of the skin and, if you choose cleverly, they can bring back light to the face via light-reflecting particles. My favourites for all three are by Dior, Laura Mercier, MAC, Clinique, Smashbox and Urban Decay. Smooth a pea-sized amount over the face, leave for a few moments, then apply make-up.

ROOT TOUCH-UP KITS

If you opt to cover grey, you're looking at a hair appointment every four weeks. Who can afford the time and money? Root touch-up kits are brilliant and buy you another fortnight between hair appointments for only a fiver or so. You stroke them along the hairline and temples and wait ten minutes before rinsing out. They come in a limited range of colours yet blend fantastically well with all. They contain PPD, though, so always patch test in advance.

FOUNDATION

It makes everyone in the world look better. I'm sorry, but it does. It unifies uneven skin tone, covers broken veins and other redness, gives a smoother base for other make-up and generally makes skin look in much better nick. Increased wrinkling can make your old foundation seem too heavy and cakey suddenly, so it may be time to choose a new one. Opt for a moisturising formula (pre- or post-menopause) to soften dry lines, or an oil-free one (while experiencing menopausal symptoms) for a long-lasting finish in the face of hot flashes. A medium coverage is most versatile, you can always mix it with a little day cream for a lighter coverage, or layer for more. (See Foundation, for application advice.)

Things that only surgery can 'fix'

Ignore the expensive product labels, the only thing that will solve these problems is a surgeon.

Hooded eyelids

These are extremely common in old age and seem to be the primary bugbear, particularly among women who enjoy beauty, since hooded eyelids restrict your make-up options somewhat. Consequently, women seem more open to spending fortunes on eye cream than any other product, but I promise they won't work. The only thing that removes them permanently is a scalpel. I'm not suggesting you go there, but it would be remiss of me not to say that an eye lift is, in my opinion, one of the more effective and subtle surgeries when performed by an expert. It is available on the NHS when visibility is affected.

Sagging neck

I receive so many emails from women asking which neck cream will fix the loss of firmness in the jawline. The answer is none. There is no way, in my opinion, that a cream can replump and refirm sagging skin permanently. The looseness is caused by a breakdown in collagen and keratin, and I don't believe that a topical cream can ever replace either (although some temporary tightening is achievable). Surgical options include thermal treatments like Accent or Thermage to re-tighten the muscle and skin (sometimes with very good, realistic results) or the more drastic surgical necklift. None of these options are cheap, or without their potential complications. But whatever you decide, you can save yourself £40–100 immediately on the 'lifting neck cream'.

DEEP WRINKLES

The only way to significantly reduce deep wrinkles is via Botox and filler, or through major surgery. See the chapter on Botox for more information on how to get them right, but before you consider it, go for a professional teeth clean and root touch-up. It's amazing how much less noticeable and/or tolerable lines become when hair and teeth look great.

VARICOSE AND THREAD VEINS

I've only recently discovered that some creams and oils suggest they might actually fix these. What nonsense. You must see a doctor if you want thread or varicose veins to disappear. Alternatively, you can apply body make-up to disguise non-troublesome visible veins. These can work brilliantly (I usually use them on my hands for photoshoots) and provided you put them on unmoisturised skin they won't easily transfer onto clothing.

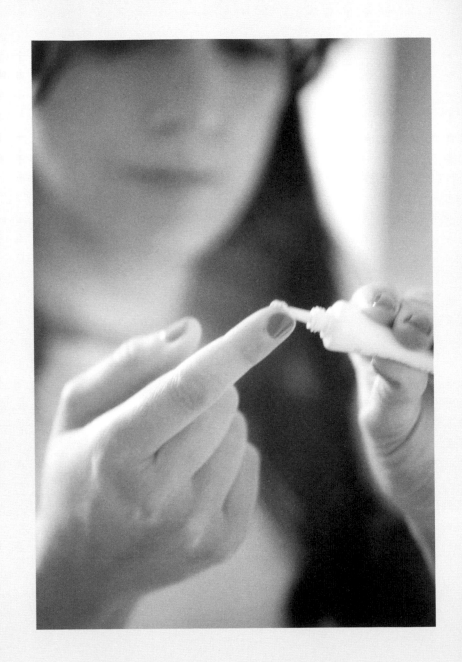

ACNE

'Zits are beauty marks.'
Kurt Cobain

People wrongly see acne as inevitable a fixture on the teenage face as the exasperated eye-roll and withering look. They may question the need to address something they simply see as an unavoidable part of growing up, but while troubles such as spots and pimples, irritation and acne are very common in teenagers, I should stress that extreme cases (and by that I mean anything that causes distress, pain or significant social anxiety) should never be dismissed as simply part and parcel of a young person's experience. They are not 'just one of those things', and teens deserve to be taken seriously. Older people often suffer from severe joint pain and mobility issues. That doesn't mean they should shrug (assuming they still can) and say 'oh well', so I don't see why young people should have to just endure chronic acne either.

I should add that it's not, of course, just the young that carry the burden of acne – incidence in adults is on the rise and most of the following guidance is appropriate to sufferers of all ages.

One of the problems with acne is how swiftly and uniformly it's diagnosed by sufferers and their loved ones. This blanket term is unhelpful in terms of finding the right treatment. Acne is a very broad church, from occasional spots (life sucks but deal with it, the health service has a lot on), to several pink 'cystic' pimples (a suitable case for treatment), to large, weeping 'pustular' sores that are purple and cover the whole face (extremely upsetting, painful and worthy of specialist medical attention). Treatment varies according to which type or types of acne you have. This is where the internet can be very helpful, if you can avoid the myriad sites that lead any physical symptom to terminal cancer requiring immediate multiple organ transplants. There are heaps of acne case-study photographs on medical sites like derm.com, which can help point you towards similarly suffering patients to gauge the severity of your own situation. If you see one that looks similar to yours, print it out, see what it's called, and take it to the doctor.

I say doctor because serious acne that is making your life a genuine drag, causing upset and depression, is a medical matter. See your doctor, ask for help and a prescription. If the treatment doesn't work, then go back and ask to be referred to a dermatologist. Many teens understandably find this sort of assertiveness quite difficult, so parents may need to get the job done.

Whether treating minor acne at home or severe acne through a doctor, the cause and management usually boils down to hygiene, bacteria and hormones (teen acne is particularly caused by increased testosterone levels during puberty). Inflammation from medication and allergies can cause acne too, though in my experience, this is more likely in adults than teens. Obviously the sensible starting point for anyone of any age is good hygiene through proper cleansing.

A teen will need to shower every day and cleanse twice (no more) with gentle, simple products that don't contain things like mineral oils and paraffin derivatives that clog pores. The vast majority of teens prefer a foaming cleanser rather than a balm or cream. I understand this need to feel 'fresh', but a face wash – especially one containing sulphates to make them foamy – simply won't help your skin. The best compromise is to use a milk or balm before entering the shower, then remove it under the water with a flannel (or a sonic facial brush if that turns them on. I am as happy with a flannel, but the best routine for teens is one they'll actually perform regularly, so any gadget that encourages use is generally A Good Thing). This method gives a proper cleanse and a 'washing' sensation without the sulphates. An evening shower may not be practical for the important second cleanse, so substitute splashes of clean tap water for shower water before moving on to other skincare.

I then recommend an exfoliant. Teen hormones can cause sluggish cell turnover and a build-up of dead skin, so removing these will help clear spots and dramatically improve blackheads (as a bonus, exfoliating is also helpful in freeing common ingrown hairs as teenage boys start to sprout facially). That said, I almost universally loathe any exfoliant which uses particles of grit to do the job. I have looked at these particles under a microscope and it's sobering. They are often so jagged and sharp that scrubbing them into skin is like being glassed a million times over. What's more, I just don't believe they work thoroughly and find they miss important nooks and crannies around the face. Those soft bead things often used nowadays in place of the grains are so completely useless I can't bring myself to say any more about them. What is ideal is a liquid exfoliant containing glycolic or salicylic acid poured onto two cotton discs and swept all over the face before moisturising.

Yes, moisturiser. I know. It may be counterintuitive to moisturise skin that is probably already oilier than is ideal, but it really is important. Products containing good-quality plant oils do not clog pores and rarely cause mischief. Many young people actively hate the feeling of oils on their skin, so a good compromise is to use an oil-free, water-based day cream to provide a nice-feeling texture and base for make-up, then a facial oil or oil-based cream before bed. This seems to keep both skin and teen happy at least half of the time. I would also suggest some good fish oil supplements – I pop cod liver oil like a nana and find it improves practically every skin complaint on record. Make sure you buy capsules, though; the liquid is absolutely repellent to you and anyone in your vicinity.

Oil-based products are still a hard sell, I know. It is tempting to starve oily skin of moisture, I really do understand. But if it actually worked, then we'd have no more acne in the world. I have never met a single case of acne that has cleared up by drying out the skin. All that happens is the complexion becomes upset, red, angry and sore. With the protective acid mantle stripped away, and with any lubrication removed by harsh alcoholic products, the skin invariably becomes very confused indeed and pumps out grease to comfort and treat itself. Either that or it becomes so uneven – horribly dry in some areas, greasy in others – that you end up with a much more complicated situation than first showed itself.

With these basics in place, you should start to see results. If not, or if your resources don't allow good skincare products, it is time to visit your doctor. That's when it gets more complicated.

In the first instance, a GP will typically prescribe peroxide skincare (often very effective) and antibiotics to treat the underlying bacteria. In my opinion, if they don't work fast (and they really can), then they're not going to and you should stop taking them. Antibiotics are simply not a long-term solution to anything. They make you feel a bit crap. Two full courses is plenty of time to give them a chance.

After antibiotics, many GPs will prescribe hormonal treatment for those experiencing severe acne. This usually takes the form of Dianette, technically a contraceptive pill but very widely used by acne sufferers of both sexes. I understand why putting a teenage son or daughter on the pill gives parents (and their teens) the willies, but it can work extremely well and I've seen great results. However, I know from personal experience that these sorts of contraceptive pills can seem to bring on uneven pigmentation problems, like those experienced by many pregnant women who develop large dark patches on their faces (called 'chloasma' and 'melasma'). These sorts of patches, while they can come and go, sometimes fading for longish spells, never completely vanish and cannot be eradicated.

Sometimes, Roaccutane is prescribed. This is not a long-term medication, it's taken in two bursts during one's lifetime, generally speaking. In my experience it works brilliantly, but it has side effects and is usually only prescribed when other medications have tried and failed.

Another very good treatment is retinol. It's one of the few anti-ageing ingredients we know definitely works, but we found this out by accident – it's actually an acne treatment. Retinols are extremely effective but can be too much for sensitive skin, causing redness, peeling and soreness. Very often though, the skin sort of pushes through the pain barrier and settles down significantly after a couple of weeks. Retinol is expensive and sometimes NHS GPs are reluctant to prescribe it, but it is available to suitable patients, so do ask. It is absolutely crucial that retinoids are used in conjunction with broad-spectrum sunscreens, as they leave skin vulnerable to sun damage.

Your last resort is paying to see a private dermatologist. The private derms I rate are all either former or existing part-time NHS. I would expect any specialist to have paid their dues by working with the broad client base, and under the strict regulations, of a public health service. I don't want a self-appointed skin doctor who has spent his entire career expertly injecting fillers. I want someone who understands how the structure of the skin reacts to burns, sun damage, cancer, injury, disease and who can take a well-rounded view with proper perspective.

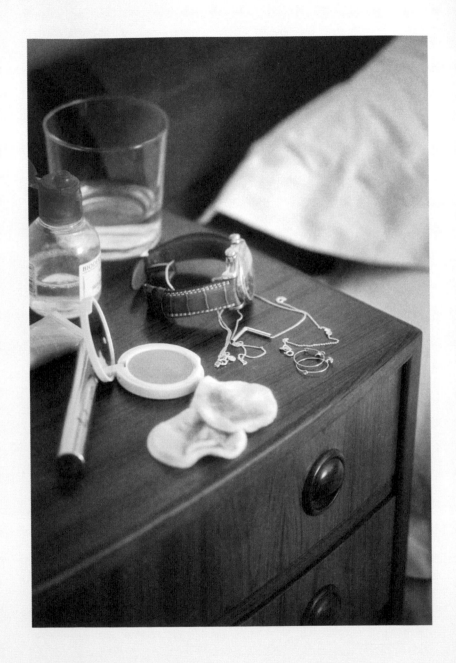

WHAT MEN WANT

'The only way I'd be caught without make-up
is if my radio fell in the bathtub while I was taking a
bath and electrocuted me and I was in between make-up
at home. I hope my husband would slap a little
lipstick on me before he took me to the morgue.'
Dolly Parton

I spend quite a lot of my professional life being asked to write about whether we wear make-up for ourselves or for men. I don't really like the inherent judgement in the question. It implies that real feminists ignore male desire on principle, and that appearing visually attractive is never a self-serving exercise but always one of piteous obligation and repression. My honest answer, after explaining that the question displeases me, is that, broadly speaking, whether or not I wear make-up is not dependent on a man's presence or wishes. It is more often for the sheer pleasure of wearing it (I love make-up – you may have noticed), or dependent on my work or female company. That is a fact, though I wish it wasn't one we women feel we have to assert constantly, as though we'd be traitors to feminism if, God forbid, we admitted we might want to look spot-free, groomed and pretty for a potential mate.

My partner sees me looking far worse than anyone else in my life. Like utter crap for the majority of the time, in all honesty. But I also like to get made up to attract him (just like I occasionally enjoy wearing a dress he favours, or decide to make his favourite chicken soup if I'd like the evening to end well). I see nothing wrong with this and I think it naive and condescending to assume it's bad and anti-feminist for women to wear make-up for a potential sexual partner's benefit. Practically every species on the planet grooms as part of the mating ritual and we all like to get laid, for heaven's sake. Make-up, for me, is one of the methods many of us women use. I feel lucky to have it at my disposal. We use all the tools we can. I knew one (bare-faced and naturally beautiful) young woman whose speciality at parties was quoting Proust at brainy boys before moving in with a killer line in 'your wife doesn't understand you' balls. How this has more honour than gluing on some falsies, I'm at a loss to say.

For me the only really important question is whether a woman feels obliged to wear make-up because of external pressures, or whether she wants to for her own free reasons. If the former, then we have a sexism problem. If the latter, and one of her motives is to get laid, then I see nothing wrong with that and people should get the hell out of her business.

So which beauty looks are attractive to men? Many men say they like no or minimal make-up, when they have little or no idea what that really looks like. When pushed for examples, they generally cite faces covered in well-applied nude shades and well-matched base as being 'bare' (this same inherent lack of awareness extends to not being able to tell the difference between a size 8 and a size 12 and being wholly unable to identify cellulite if their life depended on it. I'm extremely comforted and reassured by this). I am immediately mistrustful of men who say they 'prefer a natural beauty' because, don't we all, darling? The vast majority of us are not perfect and thus feel compelled to fake it a little. Deal with the fact that we're not all Christy Turlington and that you're lucky we're available to someone who's not Paul Newman.

That said, I know several men who swoon over a woman in bright lipstick or colourful tattoos, and others who practically get a boner when they see super-long nails painted in blood red. Each to his own. My general feeling is that date make-up should be an honest advertisement for a potential relationship. Frankly, it's easier for you that way. There's no point labouring over lots of perfectly applied make-up if you are, in reality, a low-maintenance kind of girl who can't possibly keep it up beyond the honeymoon period. Equally, it seems unwise to imply you're someone who rolls out of bed and out to a Sunday farmer's market all natural skin, flushed cheeks and a smidge of lip balm when your real life is spent in full coverage foundation and smoky eyes. Like any part of dating, it is always safer to be yourself because who can maintain a lie for long? Linda McCartney said she wore no make-up on her first date with Paul because she didn't want him to be disappointed when he saw her habitually nude face every day thereafter. She had a point.

Like many women, I swing constantly between made-up and bare-faced, so a sort of beauty schizophrenia is what any potential mate can expect from day one. There is invariably a moment early on in the relationship when they first enter my dining room (not a euphemism) and turn white as they stare in bafflement at the thousands of lipsticks, foundations, perfumes and creams spilling from dedicated drawers and struggle to reconcile this obsession with the tiny middle-aged woman standing before them, dressed in a onesie and wiping bacon grease off her otherwise bare face. If I am 'doing' make-up, I wear whatever

I want. I perhaps arrogantly assume that any man who wants to sleep with me has probably already decided he likes my style and I just carry on doing my usual thing – untanned skin, bold lips, lash extensions, pink cheeks, good base. If a man had a thing for long nails, I might try them. If he hated me in lipstick, then he'd be handed his hat and coat. When it comes to beauty, I'm flexible and experimental, never dutiful and beholden. It's my show – enjoy it as a spectator if you wish.

The morning after

I hate the term 'Walk of Shame' because when I've wandered home after a fun night with a man I've invariably felt on cloud nine – giddy and satisfied, not shameful and sheepish. Nonetheless, on these occasions I have not looked great. There have been times when, having been invited out for eggs and bacon the following morning, I've spent the whole time covering the dry, flaky skin on my chin with my hand, and hastily rubbed off smudged mascara using a fry-up knife as a mirror. An entirely spontaneous shag is hard to plan for (this is why it's good to end up in your own bathroom), but for a big date that is likely to end well, packing a small survival kit means you can extend to brunch the next morning – or even the following week. Shove it in your bag (another reason why tiny clutches are useless) and you're sorted.

THE WALK OF SHAME: YOUR BEAUTY ARSENAL

A small bottle of Micellar lotion
A super-gentle and clear lotion to remove all traces of make-up, including heavy mascara, red lipstick and eyelash glue. Just wipe over your face with cotton wool (loo paper works at a push). It leaves skin soft, not tight, unlike the bar of supermarket soap so many men call skincare. Bioderma, MAC and Avene all do travel-sized Micellars, or you can just decant your favourite into a little bottle before going out.

BB or CC Cream
The one time you'll see me recommending these multi-purpose moisturisers/foundations/sun protectants. A quick layer over cleansed skin removes the need for several different products and will make skin look clearer and more even. I prefer CCs on my dry skin, but if you're on the oilier side then a BB may work well. See the Foundation chapter for my favourites.

Mini toothbrush
For God's sake, brush your teeth. Your partner should have toothpaste for you to use – if s/he doesn't, looking good is the least of your worries. Call a cab.

Creme blush
This will make you look instantly better. Dot a little on each cheek and dab in a circle, feathering the edges. Smudge a little on your lips too, if you don't have last night's lipstick with you (you can tone a nighttime colour right down to a subtle stain by applying it with your finger). Pink suits everyone.

Mascara
Forget liner and shadow, mascara takes up very little room and is enough to make you feel effortlessly 'done'. Put on two coats by wiggling the wand back and forth to separate lashes.

Date make-up dos and don'ts

I do feel that if you're on someone else's watch it's good
manners to make your beauty routine as quick as it can be.
No one likes to be kept waiting and it's suspicious when someone
needs hours to look half decent. Be considerate and ask yourself
if you really need all three eyeshadow colours and the elaborate
contouring, or whether you can cut a few corners for the sake
of good manners and easy maintenance.

....

I adore red lips but they are not compatible with vigorous
snogging unless you both want to look like Robert Smith
of The Cure. Early dates are more safely spent in nude
shades and lipstains. Blot each coat with a tissue before
applying the next. Products like Lipcote may seem
old-fashioned, but they really do work.

....

Tubing mascara belongs in your dating arsenal. Unlike
a regular mascara, which smudges, a polymer-based
tubing mascara can easily withstand a big night out, sex,
and falling asleep in your make-up without migrating
south to your under eyes and cheeks.

....

Mineral foundation, though less glowy-looking, is perfect
for any situation in which you might sleep in your make-up,
either because you're not carrying any skincare or
because you've become more pleasantly occupied. It won't
look cakey or make you break out.

....

The idea of 48-hour deodorant is slightly emetic to me,
but this is the one occasion on which it's handy. Using it before
you go out will probably see you through until morning, without
having to top up with men's deodorant, aka the worst smell in the
world. If he's a keeper, get him to switch to women's Dove.

SIX PERFUMES THAT OOZE SEX

There's no denying that some perfumes represent the olfactory equivalent of a see-through blouse. Heady and intense, they smell carnal, inviting and a bit whorish in the best possible sense. They make a great choice for a date with someone who's on a promise – even if that's someone you've been sharing a bed with for twenty or more years.

Guerlain Shalimar

....

YSL Opium

....

Chanel Coco Noir

....

Frederic Malle Carnal Flower

....

Chanel Allure

....

Mary Greenwell Fire

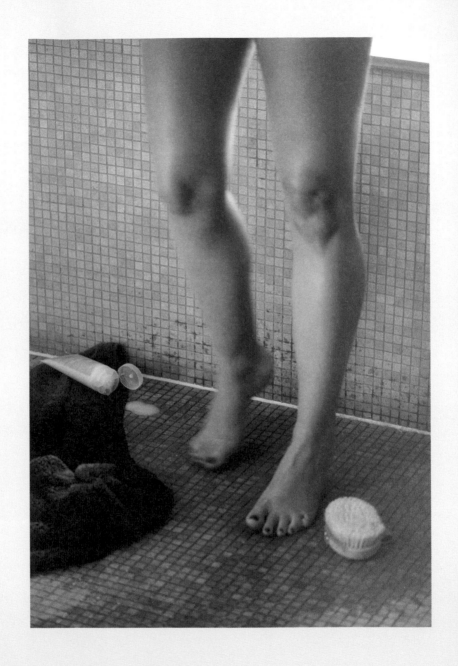

SHOWING SOME SKIN

'Even I don't wake up looking like Cindy Crawford.'
Cindy Crawford

If you're one of those women who happily wears vest tops while your smooth shoulders get darker and darker, or bares your legs as soon as the weather allows, then all power to you. If you can step out of the shower and straight into your work clothes without a 20-minute basting session with cream that feels like beef dripping, or wouldn't know an ingrown hair if it sprang from the centre of your face, then congratulations – you are winning. Perhaps your white skin turns brown in the summer and flushes healthily in the winter, or your black skin turns golden on the beach, never ashy in the cold. If this is you, then skip this chapter. What follows is for the rest of us – the women who live in black opaques and spend hours surfing the net in search of frocks with proper sleeves.

I suppose that if I could change anything about my appearance I would swap the skin on my body. I was diagnosed with a hereditary skin complaint called Ichthyosis at birth. It's a genetic condition that results in very dry skin cells that turn over and shed more rapidly than usual, causing flakiness and significant discomfort. It's high maintenance and sometimes grim, but for all the misery it caused in childhood, I've latterly come to realise that I owe my dad's dodgy skin quite a lot.

My obsession with improving my condition from the age of seven onwards caused NHS consultant dermatologists to discharge me at just 11 on the grounds that they 'couldn't do any better' than I was doing myself, and has, without question, led me down my specific career path. I was forced from an early age to 'get under' my skin, find out what makes it tick, when it responds to treatment and changing conditions and how it can be cheated into looking a whole lot better. One of the most satisfying parts of my job is having the privilege of passing on what I've learnt to fellow sufferers of problem skin, or those who have children with a skin condition they're struggling to understand.

I should say that the following is not a substitute for proper medical advice, not at all. You must ask your GP for a dermatologist referral if your skin condition is making life difficult. Truly, these men and women can work wonders and you should follow their advice. But I know from experience that most will be in agreement with me that as a long-term sufferer of any skin condition, you are your own skincare expert.

No one, including the medics, will come to understand your skin better than you will, and certainly not how to live with it day to day. Listen to what it's telling you and don't be afraid to tell your doctor when you think you know better. A good one will listen and take note.

From chronic eczema and acne to everyday dry, pasty legs or pimply upper arms, I can help you. Cellulite creams and bust gels? They can't and won't work, and I'll explain why. Don't spend another summer sweating in black opaques. I can give you skin worth baring.

PASTY WHITE LEGS / VISIBLE VEINS

Tell a person you have lily-white or blotchy legs and they'll tell you to apply self-tan – and if you can do so successfully, great. The key is to first scrub dry skin thoroughly (doing this to wet skin wastes product and works nowhere near as well), then rub body cream into dry areas that will take too much colour (knees, ankles, palms). When you've finished, don't wash your hands; you will much more effectively stop staining by massaging in rich, almost greasy hand cream then wiping your hands thoroughly on a towel you don't much care about.

If, like me, you don't like self-tan (I am literally immune to its active ingredient), then buy some wash-off tan, which in my opinion looks much more natural and is far easier to apply. The best are by Fake Bake, DuWop, MAC, Sally Hansen and James Read Tan. Start with clean, dry limbs without applying any body lotion or cream (body lotion will cause it to streak and transfer onto clothes). Apply the tan sparingly, in layers, with your hands (or tanning mitt if you prefer). Allow to dry for a few minutes before dressing. Wash off in your next shower.

ASHY LIMBS

Problem

Dark skins are prone to greyness and a dull finish, especially in winter months. Skin can look a bit like it's behind a sheet of tracing paper.

Treatment

What you need is an alpha hydroxy acid, delivered in scrub or body cream form (or even both). This will gobble away the dead cells that make the skin's surface uneven and grey. It needs doing regularly in most cases – a couple of times a week at least, if not daily. Don't make the mistake of assuming cocoa butter or another moisturiser will work as well; it will provide a quick fix by gluing down any flakes, but you'll be back to square one by bedtime.

VITILIGO

Problem

Vitiligo is a long-term condition that causes pale white patches to develop on the skin due to lack of a chemical called melanin. It can occur anywhere, but usually on the face, hands and arms. It's more common in Afro-Caribbean skin.

Treatment

Vitiligo can't be cured, but it can be disguised very effectively. Buy a specialist camouflage cream from Vichy, Keromask or Dermablend (you may be able to get it on prescription from a dermatologist). You need one that matches your darkest tones. Apply the cream onto clean skin with a sponge or brush, using a stippling-type action. Use a smaller concealer brush for around the eyes, in the creases of the nose, etc. You may need a few layers, but wait a minute or so between each. Take a loose powder, either transparent or matched to your darkest patches, and dust lightly over the make-up. You must do this to lock it down.

CELLULITE

Problem

Orange-peel dimples on thighs, bum, knees or upper arms. I hesitate to call this a problem since every woman I know has cellulite somewhere or other. Equally, I know not a single man who could identify it if his life depended on it, much less take objection to it. Nonetheless, if you want to disguise it...

Treatment

Do not buy a cellulite cream, gel or any fangled contraption for 'zapping' the dimples. I'm sorry to tell you, but in my opinion they simply cannot work. Cellulite is the outward appearance of fat cells. Nothing topical can burn fat cells. This is a nonsensical idea that is costing women billions in wasted cash. Don't get sucked into it.

If you want to improve the appearance of cellulite, the best way is to make your skin as smooth as possible through exfoliation. Get yourself a robust salt scrub for the body. You don't need an expensive one, but make sure it's not one with 'beads' in it. They are useless; you want big, rough flakes of salt. Massage the affected areas rigorously before you enter the shower. Rinse off under the water. Follow with either moisturiser or, for maximum cellulite flattery, wash-off tan (see above).

ECZEMA

Problem

Red weals and dry, sore patches on the body. Often seen on inner arms, behind the knees and around ankles.

Treatment

Sadly, there is no fix, only good skin management. You must in the first instance see your GP and get a referral to a dermatologist for expert diagnosis (there are several different types of eczema, including seborrhoeic and contact dermatitis) and appropriate treatment. If a flare-up is particularly extreme, s/he will probably prescribe topical steroids, which are very effective in the short term but should not be used for a long time as they cause damage to the skin. You'll also get emollients for washing and applying to dry skin afterwards. Having been on the receiving end of many of these prescription creams for many years, I will say that I find them less effective than great-quality creams made by non-pharmaceutical brands. This, I believe, has more to do with cost and budgetary restrictions than the genuine belief of well-meaning derms that these greasy, mineral-oil-rich lotions are actually the best thing. But that is only my opinion as a long-term NHS derm patient who comes from a pro-science and largely pro-chemical stance.

This is one of the few instances where I feel natural products can often be much more effective. What I like are shower and body creams containing avocado, olive or almond oil. These don't need to be expensive (I've bought them from the groceries section and simply poured them into simple body creams before now). I also like shea butter, which can be bought inexpensively from most high street pharmacies. All are very emollient and form a good barrier against the elements. I also like creams containing hyaluronic acid as they tend to leave skin more supple and less uncomfortable. Steam rooms can also be extremely helpful, only in short bursts of 5–10 minutes though. There's evidence to suggest than eczema patients are more likely to be deficient in vitamin E, though the jury is still out on whether supplements will help. I would take them anyway.

There are heaps of things you can do to prevent serious eczema outbreaks. One should always wear hypo-allergenic gloves for housework and washing up, avoid excessive consumption of dairy (I know, cheese. Life is extremely unfair), and use very, very gentle cleansing products, avoiding acids and retinoids. Don't swim in chlorinated pools without plenty of barrier cream and use only unscented body washes, never soap. Pure cotton clothing is less irritating than man-made fibres and stress is to be avoided, but isn't it always? Easier said than done, of course.

To cover eczema breakouts, follow my instructions for vitiligo, but be kind to your skin and give it plenty of days off.

ICHTHYOSIS

Problem

Ichthyosis is a genetic skin condition typically resulting in extreme dryness and dehydration which causes skin cells to 'turn over' either too rapidly or too slowly, resulting in flakiness and a rough, scaly appearance. The most common kind in women, Ichthyosis vulgaris, comes in varying degrees of severity, from a little dryness to seriously painful, weeping and even bleeding patches of skin. It is usually worse on the body than the face. Ichthyosis sufferers (like me) will typically have very lined hands and feet.

Treatment

Ichthyosis is with you for life, but in many cases, you can alter its effects quite dramatically. My father had a slightly milder case than mine (as does my youngest son), and yet his appeared much worse because I was so much more conscientious in treating it. The most important thing is that you moisturise every day, from top to toe. You are simply never going to be able to 'shower and go' without suffering the repercussions. Whenever you have time, use a body scrub before entering the shower (see 'Ashy skin'). Then use a rich shower cream (the prescription ones make me feel dirty and greasy), pat your skin dry, then follow with rich body cream all over your body. This takes about ten minutes after showering and is annoying, but well worth it. Incidentally, I find shaving my legs extremely helpful on ichthyosis. It removes the fine flakes on my limbs. Any shaving must be done after exfoliating, never before, and blades must be very sharp. Also enormously helpful are steam rooms for as long as you can stand them, humid climates (New York in the summer is the only time I can rush my shower routine) and creams containing hyaluronic acid (unlike with eczema, I find non-prescription chemical involvement to be essential here. I use Neutrogena and Garnier). Avoid chlorinated pools like the plague. I should also advise you to skip the long, hot baths, but I can't quite stay away myself.

PSORIASIS

Problem

Psoriasis is believed to result from a fault in the immune system. Its effect is not a million miles from ichthyosis, as cells turn over too rapidly (healthy skin cells replace themselves in 3–4 months; psoriasis suffers get new ones every 3–7 days). The result is a sort of backed-up crust of skin cells, causing itchiness, redness and soreness.

Treatment

Psoriasis is often triggered by illness, infection or stress, so keeping well is the best preventative measure. Cold weather also seems to exacerbate it so wrap up warm, wearing cotton tights (lycra seems to be fine for sucky-inny purposes), rather than nylons. Always moisturise straight after showering with a rich barrier cream. Shea butter seems to be particularly good and is, in my opinion, more soothing than prescription creams. I also think shaving with a sharp razor helps, provided the scales aren't tender and painful. To cover psoriasis scabs for a special occasion, follow the instructions for vitiligo, but begin with a coating of brow wax to create a smooth, waxy surface, available from professional stores (see Specialist Shops).

BUMPY UPPER ARMS

Problem

Bumpy upper arms (Kerastosis pilaris) are very common and are thought to be connected to poor circulation and sluggish skin cell turnover. The arms are also often red, making the wearing of sleeveless frocks a bit undesirable.

Treatment

These can be drastically improved or fixed with good, regular exfoliation. Use a good body scrub containing alpha or beta hydroxy acid before every shower in the run up to a special occasion (brides in sleeveless dresses should start several months before the wedding). Moisturise immediately after showering with an AHA or BHA body lotion or serum (Palmer's and Clarins make brilliant ones). Apply again before bed and even during the day if you can find either the time or inclination. Even out any remaining redness by stroking on wash-off tan or body make-up (MAC makes a brilliant body foundation in every skin tone, from light to dark).

BINGO WINGS

Problem

Wobbly arms not helped by weight loss.

Treatment

Do not waste your money on creams and gels that claim to tighten the skin around your arms. I believe them to be utter balls. In my opinion, they simply cannot work. The only way to tighten and tone arms is to exercise with weights. Even performing repeat lifts with baked bean cans for 20 minutes a day can work wonders. The same is true of sagging boobs. You can either weight train, get surgery, or accept that you are a woman and it's perfectly okay to not have a chest like Barbie. Do not be tempted to buy a bust gel to volumise what's already there. Frankly, I'd like to see them banned. Breasts are fat. If a topical gel had the power to grow fat cells then I suspect that the health service would use it to smear on premature babies to stop them dying. If they worked, little niche beauty boutiques would not keep the technology to themselves. Spend your hard-earned money on a nice lipstick or a good bottle of wine instead. And sleeves, always sleeves. They may be infuriatingly hard to find in the modern world, but they are chic, stylish and cover a multitude of unwanteds.

INGROWN HAIRS

Problem

Hairs that fail to emerge from their follicle, growing inwards and leaving bumps and pimples on the surface of the skin.

Treatment

Ingrown hairs are very common in women who wax and shave (and also in men). They result usually from the follicle surrounding them becoming covered with either swollen or dead skin. The way to prevent them is through proper exfoliation with a good scrub, applied to dry skin then washed off in the shower. A body lotion containing alpha hydroxy acid will also help prevent and, to some degree, treat them (though neither should be done immediately after epilation). If the ingrown hair is too set in, then you must remove it physically with tweezers. Everyone should own a super-sharp pair with a slanted edge – I favour Rubis, though Tweezerman are also excellent. Cheap tweezers are always useless and are as much good as a wooden spoon for the purpose. To remove an ingrown hair, exfoliate first and pat skin dry to avoid slip. Take the tweezers and gently scrape away the top layer of dead skin until the hair is exposed. Then, using the sharp tip, pluck – a good pair of tweezers will make light work of this. This is deeply satisfying and gratifying. Frankly, I almost feel sad when several months pass without the opportunity to perform this basic surgery.

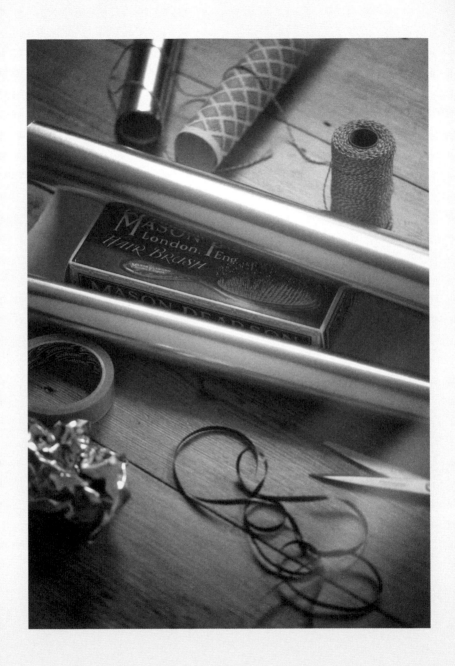

BEAUTY GIFTS

'Some people think luxury is the opposite of poverty. It is not. It is the opposite of vulgarity.'
Coco Chanel

Everyone expects me to give beauty gifts for Christmas and birthdays and it's a responsibility I've taken seriously since I was 12 and saved my allowance for months to give each of my schoolfriends a Clinique soap (for an unprecedented sum of £6). A beauty gift makes the best present, or the worst, depending on how you choose it.

My trick has always been to buy the smallest thing I can for my money, and it works every time. By that I mean spending your entire budget, whether £5 or £50, on a small piece of luxury with some wow factor – a Chanel lipstick or YSL nail polish, a posh candle or luxe lip balm, a barbershop shave or a tiny yet perfect vial of scent. This will invariably be something few women would think to buy for themselves because they cannot justify £20 on a single nail polish, however perfect and lovely, when there are nappies or petrol to pay for.

By extension, never, ever be tempted to get bang for your buck. Huge bodycare gift sets contain no more than one or two useable products, and those enormous make-up palettes containing five thousand eyeshadow shades are good for no one but a 12-year-old. Those massive, pricey wicker baskets full of crappy toiletries will go straight under the stairs or be left to gather dust and fade to yellow on the bathroom windowsill until it can be forced on an unloved houseguest who will shove it under their bed, and so the piteous cycle continues.

There are challenges, of course. You may not be confident about identifying someone's skin type, or you may feel it insulting to presume. You perhaps don't know which type of scent they wear, or do but hate it so much you don't want to enable it (frankly, I buy Kylie's Darling for no one). But some presents can be bought without insider knowledge and still make someone's Christmas. Here are some of my favourites for every occasion, from sweet sixteen to Father's Day.

Teenage girls

Skincare basics
All teens, whether male or female, are conscious of their skin. A birthday or Christmas is a great opportunity to get them started on a solid routine of cleansing, exfoliating, moisturising and protecting. Choose a routine that is good quality but not prohibitively expensive or your teen will give up when the tubes run dry. Liz Earle, Body Shop, Elemis, Neutrogena, Benefit and Clarins all make brilliant skincare for classic teen skin types.

Luxury lip gloss
Teens love gloss like I love cheese. Certain brands combine gorgeous formulas that look more sophisticated than jammy, and come in pretty, gift-friendly packaging. Pinks and peaches are reliable choices for all ethnicities. Benefit, MAC, Urban Decay and Smashbox are ideal.

Train case
This is a professional make-up artist's carry-all, containing pull-out trays for lipsticks, eyeshadows, hair grips and so on. They fulfil two functions as a gift for teens: they hold products close to hand and they help keep messy bedrooms tidy. There are hundreds on Amazon (in a huge selection of colours, prints and prices), but the best ones are often in professional make-up stores, in particular those by Japonesque, MAC and Make Up For Ever.

A proper perfume
There's a lovely tradition in France whereby on her sixteenth birthday a girl is taken to the Guerlain boutique by her mother or grandmother to choose her first signature perfume. A great perfume is a wonderful gift and choosing it a lovely bonding exercise. Clearing an afternoon to browse a department store perfumery, deliberate over tea, then buy a lovely little bottle wrapped up especially for her, is a great way to mark a landmark birthday for a daughter, niece or goddaughter.

Nail art
You may hate it, but nail art is here to stay. It's not something I engage in much but I know that if I was still in my teens, I'd be all over it like a cheap suit. Nail art can look cool and fun on the young and is an enjoyable and creative pastime. A few choice supplies – foils, line and dot pens, crackly glaze, stick-on gems and decals – from Topshop, Models Inc, Revlon, Sally Beauty Supplies or Andrea Fullerton – will go down well.

Manicure and pedicure
Most teens have never set foot in a beauty salon, never mind sat in the chair and enjoyed a treatment. A professional manicure or pedicure in a nice salon is a lovely rite of passage, feels exciting and grown up and is a nice way to get nails into shape so they can be maintained at home. It also works brilliantly as a reward for stopping nail biting.

MEN

Barbershop shave
I've never met a man who wasn't wholly turned on by the idea of a professional shave with hot towels, a tonic splash and carefully applied swirls of velvety shaving cream. Again, few could justify the cost, so the gift of a barbershop shave tends to go down brilliantly. Most towns have a grooming parlour or good barbershop these days. For the Rolls-Royce of shaves, get him a voucher for Geo. F. Trumper, barbers to the royal family (and who are not as horrifically spendy as you might imagine).

Fragrance
I adore great fragrance on a man, and in my experience most are very happy to wear it. Scent is a very personal thing, of course, but some seem to smell wonderful on everyone and can kick start experimentation with other fragrances. My favourites are Chanel Pour Monsieur, Dior's Eau Sauvage, Guerlain's Vetiver, Neroli Portofino by Tom Ford, Ormonde Man by Ormonde Jayne and Hermès Eau d'Terre.

Hand cream

I get hundreds of letters every year from men complaining of uncomfortably dry hands. Who knew? They've inspired me to give hand creams to men with great success. The trick is to choose one that isn't overly perfumed and is wholly without grease. Kiehl's, L'Occitane, Liz Earle, Diptyque and Clinique all tick both boxes.

Posh shaving products

There's a lot to be said for weaning a man off a nasty supermarket foam and onto a lovely oil-rich, softening shave cream. This is not the same as one of those old-fashioned shaving kits that most men will receive during a lifetime of Christmases. Sure, they look nice, but they probably won't get used. I love Miller Harris, Geo. F. Trumper, Kiehl's, C.O. Bigelow and L'Occitane.

Moisturiser

Not only a gift for him, but also a gift for any woman who's seen the telltale finger marks in her jar of day cream. Most men now realise that moisturiser is basically necessary and would almost certainly use one given to them. Keep things simple unless your recipient is highly sophisticated and clued up. A basic day cream or post-shave balm (preferably in a tube or pump, men don't much like jars, I have found) from Clinique Skin Supplies For Men, Clarins, Anthony Logistics, Liz Earle or Lab Series will perform well and not cost him the earth to replenish if he gets hooked.

Shower gel

Men's shower gels generally smell bad, in my experience. For everyday use, I recommend neutral-smelling, non-gender specific, shower products from Dove, Nivea or Palmolive. But for special occasions, it's nice to push the boat out for a tube of something a bit treaty. Kiehl's, Molton Brown, C.O. Bigelow, Body Shop and Liz Earle all make fresh, fruity, masculine or unisex gels and creams that men love. Alternatively, you could treat a sporty man to a relaxing muscle soak product from Elemis, Aromatherapy Associates, Thalgo or Dead Sea Magik.

Sonicare and Air Floss

To be perfectly honest, I'd argue that everyone needs a Sonicare toothbrush, but they are a reliable hit with men. A man who enjoys gadgets will like having a state-of-the-art toy to play with, a man who couldn't care less about gadgets will quite like having teeth that feel cleaner than ever. Don't confuse a sonic toothbrush with an electric one; the latter are barely any cheaper and feel nowhere near as good. If you're feeling particularly flush, get him a sonic air-flosser to go with.

Styptic pencil

Cheap as mints and endlessly useful, a styptic pencil is a little crayon drawn onto shaving cuts to stem bleeding, making those manky little squares of torn-off toilet paper redundant. They've been around for hundreds of years, but in my experience, are an entirely new and life-changing concept to most men. You can buy them for pennies at grooming parlours, old-fashioned chemists and barbershops. A brilliant stocking filler.

GIRL FRIENDS AND SISTERS

Chanel lipstick

What can I say? This is just a lovely, lovely thing encased in the chicest packaging money can buy. The solid click, the classic monochrome design, the feeling that you're in a Françoise Sagan novel every time you touch up your lips at a café table. There's nothing to not love. Red is a good, celebratory and universal option for all skin colours.

Pocket atomiser

A genius and cheap gadget that everyone should own. You simply press it down on the uncovered lid of your full-sized perfume spray and the atomiser magically fills with enough scent for about a fortnight, allowing you to travel without breakages. Travalo and John Lewis make them.

Tweezers

A really brilliant pair of tweezers is a gamechanger. You have no idea how crap most are until you own some decent ones. Rubis make my favourites, Tweezerman are also great. They will remove even the tiniest hair or the deepest ingrown quickly and painlessly. Get slanted.

Luxury nail polish

A spendy nail lacquer in a deep, jewel shade is flattering to all skin colours and a pleasure to use. A luxury brand like Chanel, YSL, Tom Ford, Dior or MAC never fails to thrill. Revlon are wonderful too. Red or burgundy are failsafe.

Candles

I adore candles, but very cheap ones are a false economy. A quality candle will burn much longer and throw scent much further, fragrancing the whole house for days. I love Diptyque, Timothy Dunn, Bella Freud, Roja Dove, Le Labo, Byredo, Jo Malone, Miller Harris and Space NK. Melt are also wonderful and much less expensive.

Empty palettes

It may seem unglamorous, but in my experience, empty make-up palettes make a very well-received gift. Start it off with a couple of basic nude shades and let her fill the rest to create a no-waste make-up wardrobe. The best are by MAC, Trish McAvoy, Bobbi Brown, Kiko, Make Up For Ever and ScreenFace.

Mums

Handwash
Everyone needs handwash, but one that smells lovely, looks nice and leaves hands soft is a rare treat. Compagnie de Provence is not too expensive and makes a beautiful gift. I also love L'Occitane, Molton Brown, Cowshed and Caudalie. All have matching hand creams.

A compact mirror
Every woman needs a magnifying compact mirror, but they become especially useful as we get older, when eyesight may be shorter. Besides, compacts are just chic and glamorous and can be bought blind as they contain no make-up to colour-match. I am never without my Chanel version, but I also love those by Stratton (my grandmother's favourite), Estée Lauder, Cath Kidston and Lulu Guinness.

Roja Dove consultation
If money was no object, I wouldn't buy a super-luxe face cream, I'd buy this, a consultation at Roja Dove's Haute Parfumerie in Harrods. While you enjoy afternoon tea, a consultant personally trained by Roja (one of the world's leading authorities on perfume and the man who personally inspired my love of scent) will guide you through an exclusive selection of perfumes, helping you find your signature scent. The wonderful Les Senteurs offers a similar service, which is also bliss.

Mason Pearson

I've given many Mason Pearson hairbrushes as gifts in the past. They're one of my favourite presents because they last a lifetime, are handmade in Britain and are useful to everyone (they even do little ones in baby blue and pink – my Christening gift of choice). They are especially great for mums, who seem to appreciate their quality and design, which is peerless. They tame thick frizzy hair and groom fine hair without causing static. They are, without question, the best brushes for drying fringes and the most adept at backcombing without tears. Not cheap, but so, so worth it.

Fragrance layering products

Most women will splurge on perfume but scrimp on body products (I'm one of them), so a matching cream or bath foam is a lovely treat. Almost all perfumes have a complementary body range. Using them gives scent more depth and longevity. Those by Chanel, Estée Lauder, Diptyque and Clarins are especially lovely.

SIX CHEAP AND LOVELY STOCKING FILLERS

*A bar of lovely soap. I like Yardley tinned soaps, classic Pears'
bars and Bronnley lemon- and lime-shaped guest soaps.*

....

*Barry M glitter pots. So satisfying and fun. Dab on eyes
or cheeks, over lip balm for sticking power.*

....

*Organic coconut oil from a health shop. A lovely moisturising
treatment for skin, nails and hair.*

....

A Kent comb. The best combs, in every shape and size.

....

*A vintage-style lip balm. I like Rosebud salve, Kiehl's Pear balm,
Burt's Bees and Perfumeria Gal Madrid. All are under £10.*

....

*An acrylic nail polish and lipstick caddy. This one of the best presents
I've ever received. John Lewis and Muji sell them.*

SOME GIFTS TO AVOID

Any anti-ageing cream unless it's been specifically asked for.

....

Ditto anything for cellulite, stretch marks, dandruff, dentures, bad breath.

....

*Pre-packed mega baskets or boxes. They beg to
be re-gifted to someone unloved.*

....

*Those manicure kits containing a metal nail file hard enough to break
out of prison. They're often bad quality and damaging to nails.*

....

*Those enormo-palettes containing dozens of shadows, blushers and glosses.
The vast majority won't get used and even if you're gifting a budding make-
up artist, the quality is usually poor. Get refillable palettes instead.*

....

Bath cubes. No one has used these since 1972.

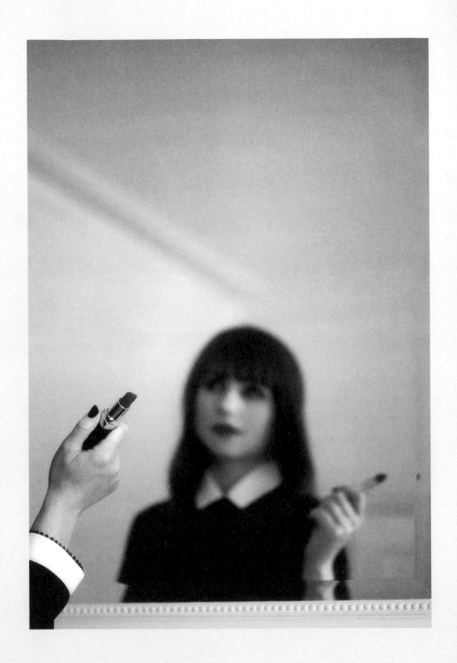

RED LIPSTICK

'Beauty, to me, is about being comfortable in your
own skin. That, or a kickass red lipstick.'
Gwyneth Paltrow

Red Lipstick is the Little Black Dress of beauty. No item sums up beauty so succinctly – if you had to imagine a make-up item, you would probably picture a red lipstick before foundation or mascara. Red is powerful, strong, smart, bold, sexy, lethally feminine and iconic (try to imagine Marilyn Monroe without her glossy, orangey-red lips – it's not possible). It moves every outfit instantly up the dress-code scale, transforming jeans and T-shirts into appropriate evening wear. It brightens the face, giving it a strong focal point and allows you to skip the faff of complicated eye looks in the sweeping of a glamorous tube. The right red makes skin appear clearer and teeth whiter. Nothing has such glamorous, timeless appeal. It breaks my heart that so many women are scared to wear it.

I've been wearing red lipstick since I was 13, when Miss Selfridge's Doris Karloff crimson gave my weekend uniform of Smiths' T-shirt, vintage Levi's and Doc Martens some much-needed femininity without compromising my then-relentlessly arsey attitude. It is probably the only part of my make-up style that has remained constant throughout my life and I know I will never stop wearing it. Nowadays, I team red with practically anything – a sweater dress on a loafing day when I need a swift kick up the backside, in important meetings when I want people to know I am not to be screwed with, at parties that deserve some effort or just on days where I need the extra backbone that red provides. I don't wear red every day – I'm too greedy to be monogamous, and besides it would make it feel less special. But there are times when only red will do. It's a cheerer upper, a motivator, a game-changer, a weapon. Red is so much more than a colour. It's a state of mind.

This is why I warn women not to obsess too much over their skin tone and hair colouring when choosing a red. Yes, finding a flattering red is half the battle, but before you can feel great in even the perfect one, you must first accept that there is a period of readjustment during which it is a mistake to flake out on grounds of self-consciousness. We are talking about two, maybe three evenings of increased self-awareness, where you wrongly assume everyone is looking at your mouth and thinking 'oooh, you're fancy tonight'; where you instinctively cover it, as though masking appalling halitosis, when all you are effectively doing is merely daring to be noticed. Please try wearing red on three occasions before making up your mind. If you still feel uncomfortable at the end of the third, bin it. But if you overcome the self-awareness, I promise you will love it forever.

HOW TO FIND YOUR RED

I am nerdish about tracking down perfect shades. Last year I interrogated someone in John Lewis about where she'd found her perfect matte brick red (Kate Moss for Rimmel) and stopped an 80-something lady behind Oxford Street to ask her about her gorgeous retro scarlet (Elizabeth Arden), then bought both the same day. But finding your staple red is really not that hard. Here's how.

As a general rule of thumb, the paler the face, the orangier the red should be. Cool, blue-based reds are more flattering against dark skins. Not that this means the very white can't look cool in blue-reds and the very black can't look amazing in orange-reds – rules are there to be broken. But it's wise to follow this basic one for your first red. You can always experiment later when you're firmly on side.

Think about finish. Lipstick is a broad church, ranging from the sheerest red tint or gloss to deep, creamy, dense matte. If you are very nervous of red, or if your work dress code forbids, then go for a stain, worn in one coat and blotted well with a tissue. Otherwise, a good first red is a satin-finish lipstick. This is neither glossy nor matte, but somewhere in the middle. It's grown up and chic, keeps lips comfortable and soft and contains enough pigment to make a statement.

Do you want a pure pillarbox red, or a more muted tone? Brick reds and cranberry shades can be very pretty and soft and are often closer to one's comfort zone than the pure crimson of a Chelsea Pensioner's coat (my preferred shade). They are good gateway reds – a few months' wear and you will probably want to go brighter.

Avoid sparkle. Frosty reds can be effective on certain party looks, but they have no business calling themselves red lipstick. A proper red has no glitter, no frost, no sparkle. If you really must have glitz, then layer a sparkly red gloss over a red lipstick.

How to apply red

If you're wearing foundation (unless you have perfect skin, red looks best with a good base), smooth it all over your mouth area and blot with powder.

....

Take a red or nude lip pencil and, starting on the top lip 'V', trace over the outline of your lips, top and bottom. Colour in the inner corners. This will stop your lipstick disappearing throughout the day. Lick your teeth.

....

Applying straight from the stick (which should be slanted, I don't understand flat lipstick nibs at all – the shape when new is there to help you. Don't spoil it), stroke the point of the lipstick upwards into the lips' V, on either side, then along the whole lips, with the pointed nib faced upwards and flat against the skin.

....

Repeat on the bottom lip, from side to side.

....

Blot with a tissue, kissing it but not moving the tissue. Reapply as above.

....

Put your whole index finger in your mouth and close your lips around it. Pull it out slowly. This will remove any bits of lipstick that would otherwise stick to your teeth.

....

Touch up every three hours or so, depending on activity (more regularly if this is of an amorous nature).

WHEN RED LIPSTICK DOESN'T LOOK GOOD

On mouths with a very thin or no upper lip.
Use a red gloss or tinted balm instead.

....

When you aren't prepared or able to retouch at least once
during the day. Worn-off red looks like you're at the end of a
big night out. It needs to look smarter.

....

With lots of dark, dramatic eyeshadow. Great in a
Robert Palmer video, terrifying and ageing in person.
Only drag queens and Joan Collins can pull this off well.

....

With tan blusher. See above.

A NOTE ON PACKAGING

Reapplication is a necessary part of wearing red. I say embrace it.
Touching up one's lipstick is a good look, especially when its packaging
is a stylish accessory in itself (see also: face powder compacts, in the
Beauty and the Careerwoman chapter). I always consider tube design
when choosing a red before an engagement. Tom Ford, Chanel, Dior,
Clinique, Elizabeth Arden, Givenchy, Guerlain and Estée Lauder all
have boast-worthy tubes that look great pulled out of a clutch at a
restaurant table.

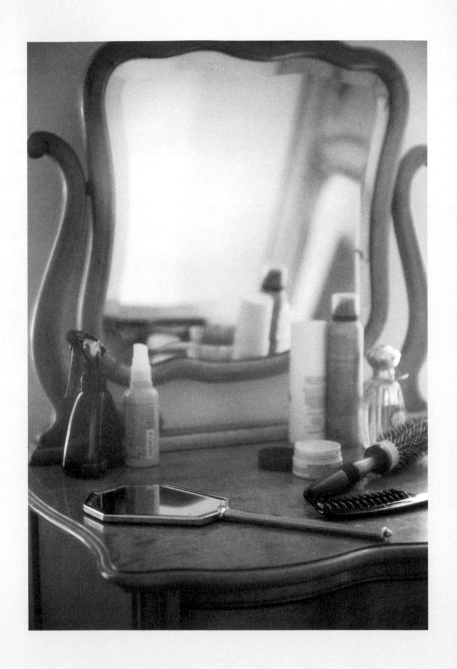

HAIR PROBLEM SOLVING

'Gorgeous hair is the best revenge.'
Ivana Trump

My hair is naturally flat and puny, growing poker-straight from a scalp that feels as though it is packed in silica gel. I'd long for curls if I didn't have so many friends locked in a furious, thankless battle with theirs (no one likes their hair. This is an indisputable truth). Instead, I've learned to tame my less-than-ideal barnet and show it who wears the trousers. I enjoy the challenge of identifying a problem (or being asked about one by a reader with entirely different hair) and learning how to fix it, either by trial and error, internet research, or grilling one of the amazing session stylists I'm lucky enough to access every week as part of my job. Here are the most common problems I've managed to solve over the years, and the most reliable solutions that are easy enough for us civilians.

Problem
Fringe won't dry straight
Fix
When hair is soaking wet, comb it straight and apply a little styling cream, spray or mousse. Then take a bristle hairbrush like a Mason Pearson and with the hairdryer nozzle pointing downwards and set at full blast, briskly brush your fringe back and forth from left to right. Be firm. Don't brush forwards. Continue the left, right, left brushing until the hair is completely dry. Your fringe will lie perfectly flat.

Problem
Fringe gets greasy throughout the day
Fix
Wash your fringe every day, even if you're not washing your hair. It's extremely easy to do when you're at the basin cleaning your teeth. Just dunk your fringe under the warm tap, lather with shampoo and rinse out. You can then shove everything under a shower cap for your shower (this works better than leaving your fringe out as that always causes leaking). If you still find it gets dirty and greasy by the afternoon, spray on a little dry shampoo. Massage in like regular shampoo to absorb the oil, then brush through. Apply hairspray.

Problem
Your hair is static
Fix
This is very common in winter and the key is to try to restore moisture and handle dry hair as little as possible. Always use a good moisturising conditioner when washing. When wet, comb hair upside down with a wide-toothed comb or special wet detangling brush, and wrap in a towel – this avoids having to do too much messing with it when dry. Apply a blob of styling cream and rake through the damp hair before blow drying or leaving it to dry naturally. Rub a tiny amount of hair oil between your palms and stroke it over the ends of the hair, avoiding the roots. If your hair is consistently static, consider investing in a silk pillowcase – they really do help.

Problem
Hair dries flat
Fix
Always dry your hair against the way you want it to fall. If your hair parts to the right, brush it over to the left while drying, or dry it upside down. It will always fall back into the usual place, but if you dry against the grain, it will do so with more bounce and body.

Problem
You can't dry hair two-handed
Fix
For many of us, that effortless manoeuvre involving a dryer in one hand, pushing against a round brush oscillating in another in perfect coordination is just too tall an order. The life-changing answer comes in the form of a rotating brush. These brushes spin at the push of a button and release hot air simultaneously, giving you a big, round blow dry with just one hand. They are brilliant. Babyliss make the best, though everyone seems to have copied them since.

Problem
Your hair takes too long to dry
Fix
Drying hair from soaking wet is a big old waste of time and unnecessarily inflicts more heat damage on your hair. The answer is to invest a few pounds in a super-absorbent microfibre hair towel. These thin, stretchy towels are invaluable if you wash your hair in the mornings and need to get out to work. I wrap my hair upside down in the microfibre as soon as I've showered. By the time I've had a cup of tea and put on my make-up, my hair is almost dry and needs only a couple of minutes under the dryer to finish.

Problem
Dandruff
Fix
Before you treat dandruff you need to find out whether it's actually just a dry, flaky scalp, or whether it's oily dandruff from an overstimulated cell turnover. Dry scalp is best treated by massaging almond, avocado or olive oil into the scalp overnight, each night for about a week, then wrapping the hair in a towel for bed. Shampoo in the normal way in the mornings using a sulphate-free shampoo. The problem should clear up and will need only a follow-up treatment around once every one to two weeks thereafter. If your dandruff is greasy, you'll need a special shampoo. The best are by Phytology and Kerastase, though it's sometimes worth trying some of the prescription shampoos. I would avoid sulphate-based shampoo thereafter. Avoid dry shampoo as it seems to exacerbate both of these problems.

Problem
PPD allergy
Fix
An allergy to PPD (a compound used in almost all permanent and semi-permanent hair dyes) is extremely serious and likely to become worse with each exposure to the chemical. The allergy will remain for the rest of your life and so PPD must be avoided at all costs. Your options are to

switch to henna or other natural dyes, though these are not as effective at covering greys. If you feel as cross about this as I do, write to the hair-colourant companies and tell them. PPD is usually found in a higher concentration in dark dyes than in blonde, so talk to your salon about going blonde or uniformly silver long-term (I will almost certainly need to do this at some point).

Problem
Tousled, beachy waves look flat and rained-on
Fix
So many women want those loose, dishevelled waves but they are wolves in sheeps' clothing – infinitely higher maintenance than they look. The secret is to dry your hair straight by tipping your head upside down to lift roots, then the right way up with a Mason Pearson-type bristle brush to smooth the top. Give your hair one final blast with the cool setting, then wait a few moments. Take a texturising or sea-salt spray and mist over the length only, avoiding the roots. Fiddle a little with your fingers to separate the surface layer. Leave to dry naturally.

Problem
Hair picks up smells easily
Fix
I only have to walk past a cooker and my hair immediately reeks of sausages. Using hairspray every day is extremely good at making hair more odour-resistant. Regular washing is obviously most effective but on many hair types – thick, coarse, Afro, sensitive-scalped – washing is a huge pain in the backside that causes frizz. Instead of shampooing, try washing with a light conditioner only, avoiding the scalp. Washing only the lengths like this is also great for preserving the day-old hair manageability many of us prefer. Hairspray to finish helps a lot.

Problem

Hair is overprocessed and breaking

Fix

Stop the heavy styling and fast. Go to a good salon, get your hair cut into an easy style that requires no flat irons or tongs, nor excessive blow drying. Ask for a semi-permanent colour in roughly the same shade as your roots. Semi-permanents are great for adding gloss and shine without further damaging unhealthy hair. As the semi-permanent fades and your virgin roots come through, you won't be able to see the join (though you can use wash-in temporaries if you get bored). Condition at every wash with a moisturising formula and give yourself an intensive treatment at least once a week. Apply a little hair oil to the ends to temporarily smooth them, giving them a healthier appearance.

Problem

Your fringe needs trimming but you can't get to the hairdresser

Fix

Approach with extreme caution. Proceed only if you are relatively adept. Before you start, clip back your hair, leaving the dry fringe loose. Comb through, and with the comb, gather the entire fringe into a flat, two-centimetre section at the centre of your forehead. Clamp it between two flat fingers at the bottom of the section, approximately a centimetre from the hair tips. Take a pair of scissors and cut upwards into the tips, naturally stopping at the fingers. Do not cut across, only upwards. When you've snipped the entire section, release your fingers and comb through, snipping away any single hairs you may have missed. Never, ever cut in a fringe where there isn't already one in place. That is a job for a professional.

Problem

Your curly hair frizzes

Fix

Avoid any shampoo and conditioner containing sulphates – they can make matters worse. When hair is wet, comb it through with a wide-toothed plastic comb and tip your head upside down before wrapping in a microfibre towel. When your hair is 70 per cent dry, work some styling cream for curly hair through the lengths with your fingers. Then do the same with a little blob of silicone-free hair oil (Kerastase, Percy & Reed and Dove make good ones). Allow to finish drying naturally (the upside-down towel-dry will have given you some volume) or, if you are pushed for time, use a hairdryer with a diffuser setting. Use fingers – do not brush.

Problem
Your roots are flat, however many products you use
Fix
You may be using too many. Just one golf-ball of mousse is adequate. Dry your hair upside down, tipping up the right way only at the end, to smooth the top. Then, take a small brush with tightly packed bristles and lift sections of hair at the crown. Gently backcomb the underside of each section, one by one. Mist hairspray onto each before moving onto the next. Finish by very lightly smoothing the top layer of hair to conceal your backcombing. Finish with more hairspray.

Problem
You want your hair to curl under but rogue sections curl outwards
Fix
Firstly, unless you have a sharp bob, having everything curling perfectly under is a bit old-fashioned and frankly too annoying to be dealing with on a daily basis. Hair that is more irregular looks softer, younger and cooler. But if this happens a lot and is truly driving you to distraction, you need a rotating air styler (Babyliss make the best). Dry your hair to 80 per cent dry with a regular dryer or towel, then, using the rotating styler, take sections of hair (just the offending ones if pushed for time) and rotate it through each one, with the barrel rotating away from you. Don't touch the sections until they are cold.

Problem
Your sweepy fringe doesn't sweep
Fix
Sweepy fringes are always fashionable, so I've no idea why it's so hard to find a stylist who can cut in a fringe that sweeps off softly to one side without having to be told to by a hairdryer. The key is to get your stylist to cut a hidden layer underneath that's shorter than the fringe's top layer. When your hair is wet it should fall naturally over to one side.

Problem
Your hair extensions or weave have begun to feel uncomfortable
Fix
It's normal to feel discomfort immediately after having extensions or a weave put in, but that should lessen after a day or two as the root tension eases off. If you are experiencing long-term discomfort, or even pain, you must get the hairpieces professionally removed and take a break of a few months at least. Hurty hair can be a sign of trauma to the follicles and can result in either temporary or permanent alopecia. Don't take the risk. Lay off the hairpieces.

Problem
You can't hold curls
Fix
Whether your hair has natural wave or is poker-straight, avoid any silicones if you want it to curl. Silicones are in lots of hair products and are great at smoothing the hair – too good, in fact. They cause curls to go flat, and fast. You can spot silicones by checking the ingredient list for any word ending in '-cone' (dimethicone, for example). You may also find it helps to skip conditioner before curling the hair. It's not especially good for it but for special occasions it does give hair more lasting hold. When the hair is damp, apply old-fashioned setting lotion before drying and curling.

Problem

Your shampoo has started to make your hair feel greasy and flat after a long time of looking great

Fix

Silicones again. It is a myth that hair or skin 'gets too used' to a product and stops responding to it. I hear this all the time but in fact it's usually that product build-up is causing the less desirable finish following long-term use. The culprit is usually silicone – brilliantly useful to begin with, a total pain when it outstays its welcome. Lose it for a while, then go back to it.

Problem

Your red hair fades fast

Fix

Red colourant fades faster than any other shade. If the maintenance is too much, you may need to reconsider your choice. You can help coloured red and natural red hair in the interim by using red-pigmented shampoos and conditioners (like Aveda's Madder Root). If your red hair is simply lacking in lustre, use shampoos and conditioners designed for blonde hair. I know this seems counterintuitive but I find blonde ranges (John Frieda's Sheer Blonde, for example) give fantastic shine and gloss to redheads.

Problem

Your hair becomes static when you come into a warm building from the cold

Fix

This is really common, even in hair that is not normally static. The warm-cold-warm-cold cycle in winter can cause your hair to look as though you've been clutching a Vandergraff generator. The solution is simple. Keep a folded-up tumble dryer conditioning sheet in your handbag. When static strikes, gently and lightly stroke the top of your hair. It will be immediately tamed. One sheet will work for several goes, too. Speaking of which...

Five un-cool hair products that work

These styling products may be outmoded, but they still do their jobs better than anything.

Styling mousse

My youth was spent with hair so full of mousse it was practically crispy, but now I know how to properly use it, I love it even more. It adds more volume than anything, helps hair to hold waves and curl and suits all hair types. Squirt a golf-ball-sized amount into your palm and work through roots with rake-like fingers. I personally avoid the hair tips as mousse can make them separate and go a bit crunchy.

Setting lotion

Like your great nana bought from the chemist for 99p. It's brilliant stuff, if a bit pest-spray in aroma. You are supposed to pour it onto sections before you curl them, but that's too messy and wasteful for me. I pour the whole thing into a travel spray bottle and mist it into almost dry hair if I'm to curl it afterwards.

Curl cream

I must give props to the Curly Girl movement online (Google it) for reminding the world how great old-fashioned curl cream is on naturally wavy, curly and Afro hair. It's a thick gunk (normally a 1950s pastel pink, pleasingly) and is applied to soaking wet hair before wrapping it in a towel. It stops frizz and retains curl without weighing down the hair. Splendid stuff – and cheap.

HEATED ROLLERS

I could not live without heated rollers. People spend forever using a host of complicated tools and volumising products to ultimately disappointing effect when just whacking in a few rollers would do the job a hundred times as well. Rollers give better and more reliable volume than anything else and are really easy to use when you know how. They used to take forever to heat (and burn fingers) but nowadays digital rollers heat in literally two seconds while remaining cool to touch. Bear in mind that the bigger the roller, the lesser the curl. For a straight, volumised 'blow dry' I insert around six large rollers, wound under the hair. It takes two minutes. Leave them to cool fully while you apply your make-up, then remove and separate the curls with your fingers. Then apply...

HAIRSPRAY

The most useful styling product bar none. Hairspray prevents static (both on hair and on tights), sets your style, helps hair retain curls, waves or smoothness and makes it more dirt and grease repellent. I am never without it, though even I have my limits. Do not, I repeat do not, spray hairspray over your face to set make-up. I heard of this trend a few years ago and am alarmed by how widespread it's apparently become. Apart from being drying and harsh on your skin, it makes it sticky and a bit immobile. Use a primer under your make-up instead.

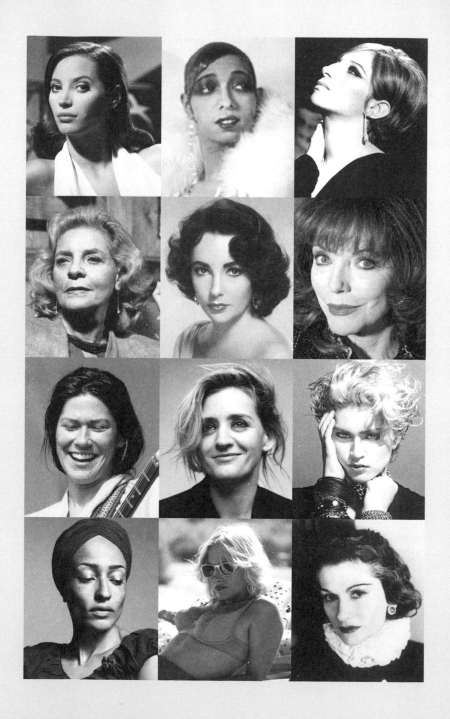

BEAUTY ICONS

'No matter who you are, no matter what you did,
no matter where you've come from, you can always
change, become a better version of yourself.'
Madonna

Everyone with even a passing interest in beauty needs an icon. I'm not suggesting a grown woman should creepily plaster her walls in posters as though a celebrity is some higher being one can never hope to be. Instead, I suggest that you look at the women around you, or in TV, film, music or politics, and identify those whose beauty inspires you to keep up your game, to try new things, to make the best of yourself and feel good about who you are. These women are diverse, in keeping with my belief that beauty is about mixing things up according to mood and self-expression – one day I might do huge Ronnie Spector eye flicks, on another I may do bare-faced Janis Joplin and give zero thought to what people say. Some of my icons are women who wear their faces proudly and uncompromisingly, others appear to have no idea how extraordinary they are. Some treat hair and make-up like a playground, using every last resource it offers to aid their creativity, others were naturally blessed in a way that seems practically immoral. I've loved some of my icons since I was four years old and still getting the same haircut as my brothers in a village barbershop. Others are new finds, reassuring me that not every ravishing beauty fits the modern stereotype of pubescent, blonde, big-titted and doll-like. I can look at my icons' faces and I feel happy, as though staring at a Henry Moore in a gallery. And then I pick up my make-up bag.

CHRISTY TURLINGTON

Original supermodel Christy Turlington, once perfectly described by fashion designer Isaac Mizrahi as 'the Sistine Chapel of faces', acts as nothing more than a source of pure pleasure and wonderment in my life. Her face is unbelievably exquisite in every way. Her cheekbones look as if they have been carved from marble then covered in pressed vellum, her lips are full and pouty in a way no doctor's injection could ever replicate, her huge doe-eyes are expressive, soulful and vibrant. I will never look like her, and that is just fine. No one will. She is a freak of nature and a work of fine art. Look at her like a rare orchid.

ELIZABETH TAYLOR

Taylor is my reminder that good grooming and glamour can be powerful, intelligent and strong. Yes, she was blessed with a natural beauty so extraordinary that one could argue (and I have) that she had the best face in the history of the world. But genetics aside, what Taylor did so inspiringly was to celebrate the overwhelming power of femininity in such a wholly unapologetic manner that just looking at her glamorous face makes one immediately feel a bit sorry for men, with their boring grooming routine and dull hairstyles. Taylor's femininity and glamour – whether embodied in a fat, thin, unwell, gorgeous or drunk as a skunk frame – were so potent they were positively lethal, never weak, meek or wasted. Elizabeth Taylor makes me deliriously happy to be a woman.

JOSEPHINE BAKER

French singer, dancer and actress Baker once said 'I have an intelligent body', which strikes me as one of the more brilliant compliments to give someone, even more so yourself. Josephine Baker, apart from being extraordinarily beautiful, stylish, talented and clever, was so, so ahead of her time. As an almost nude erotic dancer, she took charge of her public sexuality decades before Madonna was born. Her look – short hair, bold make-up and figure-hugging outfits – was modern and sexy. She was an unashamedly glamorous feminist, a proud black woman who would not bolt under pressure to conform (she refused to perform in segregated music halls and told the Ku Klux Klan, who were threatening her, that she wasn't scared of them). Oh, and she aided the French Resistance during World War II. Baker has since been portrayed by Diana Ross (another of my beauty icons) and Beyoncé, and is soon to be played by Rihanna in a biopic of her life. Ernest Hemingway described Josephine Baker simply as, 'the most sensational woman anyone ever saw'.

KIM DEAL

Kim Deal is an amazing bassist and vocalist with The Breeders and formerly of Pixies. I have a huge soft spot for women in all-male rock bands who retain their femininity in a way that in no way dilutes their tough, badass and serious attitudes (Chrissie Hynde and Debbie Harry are two of my other beauty icons who fall into this category). The first time I saw Pixies play, I realised halfway through that I had been fixated on Kim Deal's beautiful face since the first chord. Her adorable pixie-crop haircut is perfect. Her bones are exquisite and prominent, but her face is warm, soft, friendly, joyful and extremely sexy (ask any indie boy about Kim Deal for proof of its powers). She is mostly make-upless and always looks fabulous, inspiring me to hold my naked face up high. She is one of those women who is naughty, happy-looking, twinkly. Though still only in her early fifties, she is showing all the signs of being on her way to becoming the most gorgeous old lady.

ANNE-MARIE DUFF

British actress Anne-Marie Duff's face takes my breath away. Her combination of angular bones, huge eyes, small mouth and milky white skin is wholly unique, even a little strange and ethereal, but is so unbelievably lovely that I can gawp at it for hours. Despite being so distinctive looking, she is such a brilliant actress that her face is instantly believable as that of another. It emotes in a way that is completely absorbing. It's also one of those faces that makes the perfect canvas for experimentation with make-up – I suspect it can handle a faceful of greasepaint and still hold its own. I don't know Duff at all, but I always think she looks like someone who doesn't know how stunning she is, which I find charming and human. She has the sort of face that isn't particularly noticed at school, but which develops into something completely unforgettable later on.

ALABAMA WHURLEY

Alabama Whurley is not a real person but the lead female character in the film *True Romance*, played by the radiant Patricia Arquette. Her hair is pop-blonde in cheap pageant-girl flicks, her lipstick a pillarbox red, her ripe, sexy body poured into lurid-coloured spandex. She is the purest embodiment of how beauty can just be FUN. Alabama inspires me to sometimes get things a bit wrong in order to look right, to think the best taste must have a little bad taste to make it interesting.

ZADIE SMITH

Another Christy Turlington to stare at like an oil painting, dribbling slightly. I saw writer Zadie Smith in the ladies' loo at a party last year and was immediately struck by how life is so terribly unfair. I expect this happens a lot to people meeting her for the first time. Her skin is flawless and usually make-upless. Her hair always seems scraped back or wrapped in a scarf as though she can barely be doing with it. She is usually in thick-rimmed spectacles. I hesitate to say she is perfect-looking because that almost sounds pejorative and makes her seem boring-looking, when it is quite the opposite. But really, she is more pretty than a person really has a right to be.

COCO CHANEL

I adore Coco Chanel for many reasons. Dodgy politics aside, she was an awesome and inspiring woman. She (who, frankly, was not a classic 'looker') shows that being beautiful is really not about being pretty, except in the most pedestrian sense. It is about being elegant, stylish, strong, groomed, smart. She was stunning, obsessed with the pursuit of making other women look and feel exquisite and comfortable when male designers had them boned and corseted until they could barely stand. As a beauty innovator, she is peerless. She invented the suntan as a desirable state, and when she approved formula No5 from a line-up of scent samples, practically invented modern designer perfumery.

BARBRA STREISAND

Oh my, Barbra's beauty is phenomenal. And the most inspiring thing about it is it's entirely its own boss. In an age where looking Jewish and also a bit odd would have otherwise been the kiss of death to any showbiz career, Barbra emerged as one of its great beauties without having ever attempted to blend in via the plastic surgeon's office or make-up artist's chair. With long and deep-set almond eyes, a strong ethnic nose, angular bones and a wide, highly vocal mouth, she is proof that being beautiful is not about looking like everyone else, it's about looking like you on your terms. She also looks absolutely amazing in good make-up and has revelled in using it throughout her career. Today, in her early seventies, she is still absolutely breathtaking.

JOAN COLLINS

I once saw Joan on TV talking about ageing. Her fellow panellists were advocating toning things down, wearing less make-up, cutting their hair and keeping things natural and tasteful. When it was Joan's turn, she said, 'You need to wear more make-up.' While for the most part I think you should age however you see fit, I find Joan's refusal to follow the rules and to stick to her high-maintenance approach to beauty endlessly inspiring. A couple of years ago I visited Joan in her London apartment to interview her for *Red* magazine. She is, without question, one of the most beautiful women I've ever seen – at any age. Her skin, having been meticulously shielded from the sun for over 50 years, is astonishingly good (and apparently untouched by surgery). Her make-up, applied by Joan herself in ten minutes flat, is immaculate, dramatic, glamorous – all bold lips and smoky eyes. She exudes radiance and the kind of good health one prays for in old age, while admitting to all the hard work put in to achieving it. But the most significant contributor to Joan Collins' youthful look is her girlishness. She's really naughty and funny, she's sexy and playful, she loves food, men, life. And anyone can aspire to that.

LAUREN BACALL

Hollywood icon Bacall is my proof that with good bones you can never not look fabulous, however many Martinis, fags and shags you enjoy. Her amazing elderly face, no less beautiful than her young one, looks like a road map of a life lived to the fullest – every crowsfoot the sign of a laugh at a dirty joke; every sunspot a footprint of an amazing holiday with Bogey; each wrinkle an indelible marker of extraordinary experience. Her visibly Jewish face (even after a studio-enforced nose job) is ethnic, clever, wise, stylish, elegant. I love that even in her eighties she wears her lipstick dark and her hair long (I am very much against the accepted wisdom that older ladies should cut off their hair, as though they must now start to take up less precious space in the world. Ugh). Her brows are the best I've ever seen, especially when arched menacingly at chat-show hosts who dare to attempt to outwit her. She is too, too fabulous.

MADONNA

My first, my last, my everything. You don't need to love Madonna (well, you slightly do), but you must give her props for being the woman who has sucked every last scrap of marrow from beauty. Truly, no one has harnessed the transformative powers of hair and make-up to such an extent. She inspires me to constantly experiment with new looks and reference points, not giving a damn whether some people think that someone my age should settle into a life of sensible haircuts and rose lipstick. And the genius of Madonna is that whether she's wearing a black geisha wig and bright white face paint, or dark, androgynous 1920s eye make-up, cropped bleached hair and stuck-on gold teeth, she only ever looks like Madonna, never anyone else. She is also the ultimate embodiment of a woman who was not born conventionally beautiful, but absolutely sees physical beauty as her right. She does the best with what her genes gave her, as we all should.

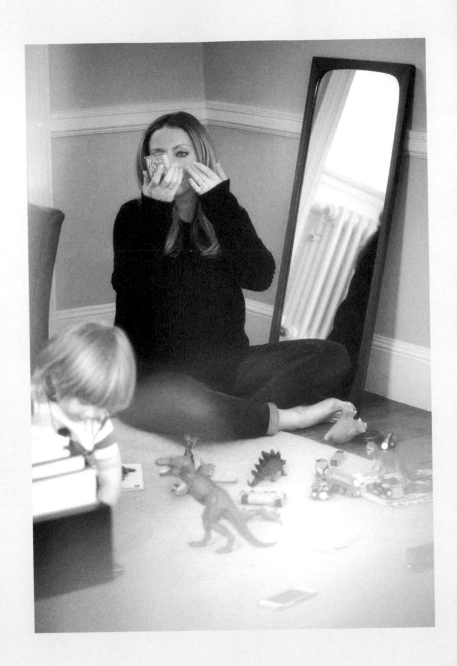

BEAUTY AND MOTHERHOOD

'Motherhood has a very humanizing effect.
Everything gets reduced to essentials.'
Meryl Streep

I felt and looked great during my two pregnancies. After the first knackered, nauseous trimester, everything seemed to take on a slightly superhuman quality. My fine hair felt abundant and bouncy, my skin, more balanced, unfeasibly smooth and perky looking. And as is typical, any neuroses about my figure vanished as soon as I stopped looking like I'd piled on burger-weight and started looking very definitely with child.

The Goddess months turned out to be a cruel dupe by nature that left me wholly unprepared for how absolutely appalling I'd look after my first baby was born. Truly, I looked instantly crap. Glowing skin became dull, even spotty for the first time in my life. My complexion was horribly dehydrated from around the clock breastfeeding and grey from insufficient sleep. What seemed like handfuls of my lovely new hair fell out onto the floor of the shower on the rare occasion I could manage one between baby naps. I wore a brown butterfly mask across my nose and cheeks where my hormones had sent skin pigmentation haywire. I smelled permanently of soured breastmilk, and felt as though I had just seconds a day to make myself presentable. Any deluded ambitions I had of scaling down to softer, low-maintenance make-up and making hair styling fashionably carefree were soon downgraded to whole days without even washing my face in case the sound of running water woke up the baby.

Yes – if you are wondering if I had post-natal depression – I was not a well girl. But mentally fit or not, I know few women who've really felt physically confident after giving birth to their first baby, which is ironic, given what feats the body has just achieved. These feelings have a great deal to do with the enormity of physical and hormonal change, of course. But I also think the post-partum period is the most acutely disorientating time for a woman's personal identity. Mourning for my career and social life, I didn't know who I was after my first baby and so I didn't really know what to do with the one thing I had always instinctively understood about myself: my appearance.

My husband was very happy and encouraging and certainly didn't feel let down by my appearance. Others were either kindly ignoring of the fact that I looked so different, or didn't notice. But other women who know the very bones of me knew something was amiss, as they so often do. For example, one girlfriend visited when my eldest son was four weeks old. Determined to demonstrate that all was well, that I was coping admirably and nailing this whole mum business, I placed the baby on a towel on the bathroom floor and blow dried my hair, put on make-up and picked out a suitable outfit. My friend and I sat in my flat, drinking tea while she cooed over my son and I said all the right things and pretended to breastfeed adeptly. It was only when she left and I was preparing to close the shutters and burst into tears again that she sent me a text from the bus, saying she'd return tomorrow as clearly something was very wrong. Why? Because I was wearing a pastel-coloured jumper from Boden. She was right. I had worn pastels for the first time in my life because I thought they'd help me get into character. After decades in heels, skinny jeans and killer make-up, I was (wholly cluelessly and somewhat condescendingly) trying to be someone else, someone who looked like a proper mum. That horrible, embellished, peppermint-green tunic had blown my cover with someone who knew me far too well.

This sort of sudden onset identity crisis is problematic. Because while a new mother may be feeling a little lost and even bereft for her old life, she has practically no time nor much inclination to chase it. The other issue is how utterly invisible women are often made to feel simply because they've given birth. I once sat around a table at a winter wedding reception with my newborn baby on my lap. I watched with some bemusement as another woman went around the table, asking each and every person on it what they did for a living – 'Oh! A nurse! How interesting!', 'Project management! Tell me more...' and so on. When she'd finished with the man to my right, she skipped straight past me and onto the person on my left. Why would I have a job, a career, or anything interesting to say, when I was now visibly 'just a mother'? It was as though she couldn't even see me – particularly gutting when I'd just shoehorned myself into Spanx and done my first flicky eye in months especially for the occasion. Some justice was done later when I stood next to her at the ladies' basins and she asked the woman on her other side if she had any make-up, as she'd left her toiletries bag in her room, but didn't bother asking invisible me. To quote Pretty Woman: big mistake. HUGE.

While I'm not suggesting for a moment that you try to win the approval of similar morons, I am recommending that if you feel as though you are losing your old self during the post-partum period, then hair, make-up (and clothes) can be a good way of keeping a grip on her while you find your way. The acts of putting on make-up, or shaving one's legs, can feel familiar when everything else seems unrecognisable. If this is the case, the important thing is to combine looking like your old self in the time your new schedule allows.

Of course, if you are either enjoying currently, or are about to embark on, your first ever period of tits-out, pyjamas-on, make-upless slobbishness and are thoroughly looking forward to it, then do please carry on (I found I was able to enjoy this part second time around, when I felt a great deal more competent and happy). To some women, the post-partum months are a gift from God, a relaxing holiday from any expectation to look effortful and to focus solely on being a parent. If this is you, please continue to do as little grooming as you please and enjoy your time. But if, like I did, you are feeling somewhat at sea and in a state of unintentional disrepair, here's some advice on how to bounce back.

COMMON POST-PARTUM BEAUTY GRIPES

CHLOASMA

These are dark patches of skin that develop during many pregnancies (including both of mine), commonly in the shape of a large butterfly down the nose and across the cheeks and temples. They can affect women of any race and often disappear by themselves after birth. However, often they don't, in which case they will probably come and go forever (mine fall into this category). Chloasma can be extremely upsetting and there is no cure. Serums and creams for fading dark patches won't help, as they are designed for hyperpigmentation from sun damage and ageing, rather than from malfunctioning cells, which is what causes chloasma (also called melasma). Some cases respond well to expensive peels and laser treatments, others don't. The safest management is with high broad-spectrum sun protection (sun aggravates the problem) and camouflage creams – the best are by Keromask, Kevyn Aucoin and Vichy Dermablend. Taking some contraceptive pills can also cause melasma.

DULL, DEHYDRATED SKIN

This is extremely common and usually comes from a combination of corner-cutting skincare (i.e. being too knackered to cleanse and moisturise before bed), not enough water (particularly while breastfeeding) and grim sleep deprivation. The solutions are obvious but easier said than done. You may find it helps to do your nighttime skincare routine much earlier in the evening, when you're slightly less tired – perhaps if your partner is bathing the baby before bedtime. Use a moisturiser containing hyaluronic acid to retain as much water in the skin as possible. Invest in a nice one-litre water bottle (Sigg make lovely ones) and make sure you empty it twice a day – it's easy to lose track of small glasses. I decided that I'd have a swig and do my Kegel exercises every time I sent a text message. If you're also an iPhone/Twitter/Facebook/Instagram addict, this may well help. Sleep is the hardest to do. I found it maddening when people told me to sleep when the baby slept, as though I didn't have a million other things already vying for the time – pumping milk, washing pukey onesies, showering, going to the loo. I am a huge believer in partners doing a dream feed at around 10:30 pm so you can go to bed at 9 or so, but also, devoutly, in facial oil, concealer and blusher – these make up the holy trinity of sleep fraud.

ACNE

Acne is usually related to hormonal change, meaning new mothers are particularly susceptible, either during or soon after pregnancy, or when stopping breastfeeding. This period can be fleeting (around three months usually) and the most effective treatment is through good skincare. (See Acne for more on the best approach.) This also commonly occurs after coming off the contraceptive pill. Again, it should settle after about three months.

SAGGING BOOBS

I mention tits because I'm desperate to share a recommendation with you. Those who tell you to always wear a soft nursing bra when breastfeeding are, in my experience, in possession of the kind of small pert boobs that don't look absolutely bloody awful in one. Mine do, and these terrible things made me feel more self-conscious about my appearance than anything else. And so I went on a mission to find an alternative. Anita is an American company that makes underwired nursing bras – comfy, non-metal, cup-unhooking, well-fitting and flattering bras that stop your boobs grazing your belly button and make you feel a half-decent shape. They are brilliant and I recommend them to anyone over a C cup. They don't affect your milk supply or feeding experience and can be found on eBay and specialist lingerie sites.

HAIR LOSS

After giving birth if bottle feeding, or later on after stopping breastfeeding, the lovely extra hair you retained during pregnancy will fall out. It's a bloody pain but absolutely par for the course. On the bright side, your hair will not, in all likelihood, be any thinner than it was pre-pregnancy, it just seems a particularly mean shot when you've got used to having masses of it. You are mostly going to have to run with it, but you can bulk up the strands with dry shampoo or hair powder, and by drying it upside down (this isn't a time-consuming blow dry, it's easy and fast). You will find wispy strands grow at your temples, almost like a mini fringe of regrowth, which you can disguise by asking your stylist to cut in a real fringe by bringing forward more hair from the crown.

STRETCH MARKS

I'm not convinced by the belief that daily moisturising with oils and butters prevents stretch marks, but it certainly won't hurt. I personally feel that if you are going to stretch, it will happen whatever you do. I do believe existing stretch marks can be treated with some success, however. If yours bother you (mine don't), then treat them by pricking open a vitamin E capsule and massaging in the liquid. Alternatively, but less cheaply, there's Bio-oil (very good) or Decléor Prolagene gel (excellent). Pale skins respond best to this treatment. The important thing with all three is to do it daily. Frankly, I could not be bothered and ended up forgetting the marks were there.

PRE-LABOUR TREATMENTS
WORTH CONSIDERING

A SWEEPY FRINGE

Fringes are high maintenance and need to be washed every day. Not having anything going on at the front makes shoving hair back in a ponytail (a staple when you have a baby to look after) a bit drab and harsh-looking. Sweepy fringes are much less hassle than the former, but add some interest where the latter lacks it. And, if cut properly, they fall into place without blow drying. Ask your stylist to give you a side parting and put in a long fringe, but to cut the under layer shorter than the top. This makes it fall automatically to one side. It's brilliantly convenient.

WAXING

I know lots of women get bikini waxes in advance of labour and if you normally wax and feel happier that way, then a good time to do it is a week before your due date. You might as well get a leg wax while there, since you probably won't be able to bend down to shave any more and may well not feel like doing anything after the baby comes. But I do feel duty bound to tell you that however you feel now, and however important this stuff normally is to you, you simply will not care about the appearance of your pubic area while in the throes of labour. I promise. You and dignity will part company the moment you're checked for dilation and may not reunite for up to 36 hours, pubic hair or none.

ROOT TINT

If you dye your hair then get your roots done as you approach your due date or, better still, consider tinting your hair to something closer to your natural colour so that undyed roots aren't visible from space. Ignore people who lecture you about the dangers of hair dyeing to your unborn child. Their information is literally 50 years out of date and they should a) get their facts straight, and b) mind their own business. You are completely fine to continue dyeing, provided you keep up regular skin testing, as anyone should.

GEL PEDICURE

No one needs this, of course, but it's an extremely cheering thing to do during the tedious final weeks of pregnancy, when you can no longer paint your own toenails and you are experiencing your last spell of self-serving pleasure. It's worth getting gels here, as they will remain perfect for a good month or so and will give you something nice to look at when you're sitting in a chair at 4am, unable to put on the telly for fear of waking the baby.

PRODUCTS WORTH BUYING BEFORE THE BIRTH

FACIAL OIL

I'm a big believer in facial oil anyway, but it is exactly the right thing for new mothers. A good plant oil nourishes and moisturises the skin, brings back glow, is unlikely to irritate the newly sensitive, smells lovely and, crucially, can be applied quickly at night in place of separate serums and night creams.

I like Neroli by Decléor, Blue Orchid by Clarins, Rosehip by Trilogy, and many others. Incidentally, it is worth moisturising your perineum with an oil in the run up to labour. Avocado oil (cheap from supermarkets) is ideal.

CC CREAM

These are ideal for new mums, as they moisturise, give good sun protection, slightly even out patches of chloasma (the dark patches of skin caused by hormonal changes) and provide fairly decent coverage.

The best by a mile are made by Origins, Darphin, Smashbox and Clinique (the latter has them for all skin tones).

CONCEALER PEN

Concealer makes everyone look better, especially the sleep-deprived. Invest in one now that is fast and easy to apply and is as good at covering spots as it is at disguising dark circles. In my book that means a wand or a clicky pen applicator as opposed to something that needs brushes, and something with plenty of coverage and creaminess. I always use either Clarins, Nars (available for most skin tones) or By Terry, but I also like Estée Lauder, L'Oreal Paris and Lancôme.

DRY SHAMPOO

Or mother's little helper... This product was made for post-partum beauty. It performs two functions brilliantly. Firstly, it allows you to freshen unwashed hair when time is tight. Secondly, it pumps up lank hair that's been left to dry naturally, giving the illusion of a semi-decent blow dry. It also comes in tiny nappy bag cans, usefully.

Everyone seems to make them now. The best are by Batiste, Trevor Sorbie, Klorane, Superdrug own label and Oribe.

DUAL LIP AND CHEEK CREME

A pretty pink, red, peach or nude shade that can be rubbed hastily onto cheeks and lips to stop you looking dead – even if you feel it. These come in a compact or stick (either is fine) and dispense with any need for brushes. They also avoid having to choose which lipstick goes with which blush.

The best are by Stila, Becca, Revlon, Tarte and Bobbi Brown.

Rich lip balm

If you're breastfeeding, you will find your lips can easily become dry as your body drains your skin of water. It is obviously very important to drink a great deal more water than usual during this time, but you can also keep lips moist with a good balm made from natural plant oils rather than paraffin derivatives. Lip balm is also very useful as a nipple balm should things become sore or cracked.

I like balms by Korres, REN, Decléor, Body Shop, Clinique, Dr Lipp and Sisley.

A new perfume

Smells that you absolutely adored before pregnancy can suddenly make you gag for no good reason. Take it from me, the negative association will probably never leave you – I still have to leave the room whenever I smell Chanel Cristalle, which is tragic as my pre-motherhood self knows it to be beautiful. Use this as an opportunity to treat yourself to a new perfume that your pregnancy nose likes, for use afterwards. A perfumer once told me that if you like a smell when pregnant, your baby won't be distracted or offended by it when s/he's born. Superstitious, unsubstantiated cod science, certainly, but I like the idea nonetheless. (See the chapter on perfume for where to go.)

A FIVE-MINUTE FACE

After your shower, comb your hair upside down and,
still bending over, wrap it in a towel.

....

Apply a hyaluronic acid-rich serum if you can, and moisturise with
a CC cream in either your exact skin tone or half a shade darker.

....

Dot the concealer straight from the packaging under the eyes
and onto blemishes, then pat with your ring finger to blend.

....

Take a dual lip and cheek colour and dot onto the fat part of your
cheeks with your middle finger. Use a clean finger to blend into
a comet shape. Use your ring finger to dab more onto your lips.
Apply a little lip balm over the top.

....

Looking down into a mirror, lift up your eyelid with your thumb.
Take a black, curling mascara and wiggle the wand from the inside
root to the tip, using a zig-zag motion. Do your lower lashes without
picking up more colour from the tube, then repeat on the other eye.

....

Let down your damp hair and spray in volumising spray to the
roots (if straight) or apply some non-silicone hair oil to the lengths
(if curly). Comb the front to the side, or blast the fringe with a dryer,
leaving the rest to dry naturally.

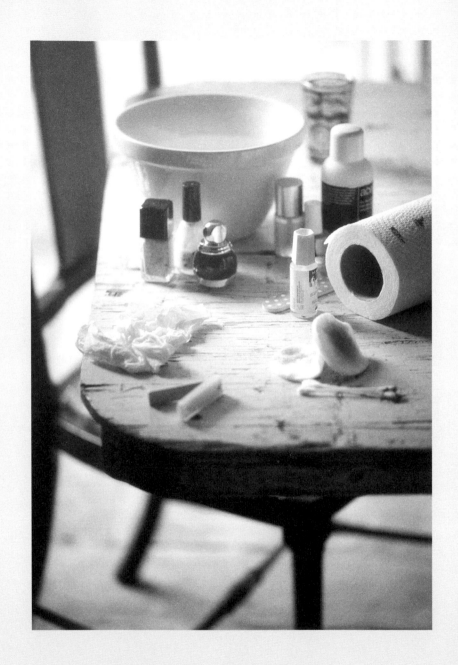

GETTING THE PERFECT MANICURE AND PEDICURE

'A woman is helpless only when her
nail polish is drying and even then, she
could pull a trigger if she had to.'
Unknown

Nails represent the biggest beauty trend in recent years. Nail art, salon paint jobs, gels, acrylics – the choice is dizzying and, to many, completely baffling. Even I, having been born with the ugliest hands in Britain, came late to the party (fancy nails were for Alexis Carrington Colby, not the asbestos-handed great granddaughter of a South Wales blacksmith).

I'm glad I caught on. Relatively easy and quite therapeutic to apply, nail polish is one of the most cheering beauty products because it instantly changes your look in a way that's wholly unreliant on the wearing of other make-up or nice clothes, or even on dragging a brush through your hair. You can be looking essentially like a pig in every other regard and yet still, every time you glance down at your hands typing a report or scrubbing the bath, there are your coloured trotters all chipper and pretty. They're uplifting.

Painted nails are also risk-free. They suit everyone, are easily changed or reset, and even women with absolutely no instinctive sense of colour or style would be hard pushed to choose the wrong shade – unless it's pink with bright white tips. (I'm sorry, but French manicures are absolutely not invited to join the twenty-first century. I daren't even think about French pedicures. I'm shuddering as I type.)

I paint my natural, short fingernails once or twice a week. They chip after about three days, then I either replace or leave them bare for the next three or four after removing (always do this when your mani gives up the ghost. No polish is, without exception, better than chipped polish). As for my toes, I don't think they've been unpainted for about 25 years. They are the only feature I never unmask and I confess to being faintly horrified when I see gnarly, unpainted toenails on Brighton beach. I can't see why you wouldn't paint toes when it lasts for several weeks (if I never got bored and left my pedi to its own devices, it would probably grow out).

So how to apply nail colour? I look at Instagram (which is wonderful for any beauty fan – do join) and despair at the paint jobs on display by those who claim to know what's what. Pools of varnish settled into nail beds, smears on fingertips, cuticles so husky and dry they look like dead moths. I often think my six-year-old could do a better job (incidentally, small boys and girls love painted nails, in my experience. A rainbow mani and pedi is a mutually diverting way to kill an hour on a rainy half-term afternoon). The blame for terrible paint jobs can almost always be laid at the doors of Too Much Paint, Too Little Time and Too Much Trying To Follow Your Own Nail Shape. I appreciate the latter is baffling, so allow me to explain.

How to paint your nails neatly

This is not a proper manicure nor a pedicure; proper manis and pedis are essentially skincare treatments for hands and feet. Lovely if you have time, or plenty of money, for a salon treatment (if you live in Britain, at least, where this costs a relative fortune) but they're scarcely a necessity. What follows is a paint job, a polish maintenance, something many of us perform once or maybe twice a week. It's the technique I use myself and, with practice, is extremely easy and causes extreme smugness and gratification. Before you start, choose a 60-minute TV programme to watch while you paint your nails – if it's on every week and can be permanently assigned as your weekly 'nail time', then all the better. This seems to be the only sure-fire way of avoiding going about your business too soon after painting and suffering the maddening smudge (on the same tip, lay out any snacks now. I enjoy a 1970s-style crescent of crisps to avoid dipping my wet nails into the bag). I find BBC's *Question Time* to be the best nail programme as it's the right time length and I don't need to be looking at the screen intently, only listening (this improves the viewing experience quite drastically, in all honesty).

REMOVE OLD POLISH AND WASH HANDS
I personally favour the quick dip-in pots of remover for fingernails, and cotton wool discs soaked in regular remover for my toes. After removing all polish thoroughly, rinse off any residue but don't follow with hand or foot cream.

CLIP AND FILE NAILS

Nail clippers are old-fashioned, but they are absolutely the quickest and neatest way to shape nails and people are mad to ignore them. They must be sharp and of good quality, not of the from-a-Christmas-cracker variety (I only use clippers from Muji, who do two versions, for fingers and toes). Sharp clippers will leave nails so clean-cut that very often filing isn't necessary, but if it is, always use a flexible emery board, not a metal file, and file across your nail tips in one direction (not in a back and forth sawing motion). In either case, you should ideally shape your finger and toenails with a square edge. It's perfectly fine to want pointy fingernails, but it's more of a faff and this technique is about ease.

APPLY BASECOAT TO FINGERNAILS AND TOENAILS

You can be relatively slapdash about this, since basecoat is clear. But don't apply too thickly as you want it to dry fast and provide a good grippy foundation for any colour. If you want to treat your nails, now is the time to do it by choosing a base coat with either hardeners or ridge filler.

COLOUR

Choose two colours. One colour on all four extremities seems a wasted opportunity and is a bit naff. In general, one can go a bit madder with toenail colour, since painted toes aren't always on show and are, in winter, largely for one's own amusement. My two colours can be anything – hot pink and red, navy and orange, purple and emerald green, glitter and matte, glossy and metallic. There are really few rules here. I think my only strong aversions are to frosty pastels (lilac creme = pretty, lilac frost = revolting). If you are not particularly adept at painting, choose a brand with wide brushes, like Essie, L'Oréal Paris, Dior or YSL. These are much easier to wrangle.

PAINT FINGERNAILS

Remove your brush and stroke it on either side against the neck of the bottle. The brush should never be dripping. Use it to paint three strokes – left, middle, right – in the shape of a nail. Do not attempt to follow the shape of your own nail bed here. Seriously, disregard your natural nail shape and stay clear away from its boundaries. There will be small, unpainted gaps between the sides of your nail and your skin. This doesn't matter. It will look much neater in the long run. Don't worry too much about any streaking at this stage. This coat is for colour density, not neatness. Leave to dry for a few minutes, then repeat the exact same process with the other colour on your toenails.

SECOND COAT

Again, it's important you scrape off the excess paint on the side of the bottle neck, but this time you can leave a little more on the brush than before. Repeat step five, but take great care not to streak. Stick to the shape you painted with the first coat and go nowhere near your nail beds, leaving a little gap all around the edges of the polish. The little extra polish should help you achieve a smooth finish, as will moving fast. Don't go back and paint over wet polish you've just laid down, if you think it's really needed, you can do it with an optional third coat.

Wait a couple of minutes, then repeat on your toes with the other colour.

TOPCOAT

After a good 10 minutes, apply clear topcoat, either matte or shiny, as you like (if you don't wait until your coloured polish is dry, the topcoat will become discoloured in the bottle). Fast-drying topcoats are great if you really are in a hurry to leave the house but I strongly believe they shorten the lifespan of your manicure and so should be used only when really necessary. This time, you are taking the varnish over the edges of the polish, towards your nail beds. This seals it in, like placing Sellotape over a narrower piece of paper. Leave a few moments and repeat on your toes.

CLEAN UP

Using a nail corrector pen (easiest) or a cotton bud dipped in remover (fine), remove any stray polish from your skin, taking care not to allow it to touch your new nails. Relax in front of the TV for at least 20 minutes before moving.

TREAT

When your nails are completely dry, slather on lots of rich hand cream, working it into the cuticles. You can follow with oil before bed (it's worth doing this every night before sleep).

Nail SOS

Nails are on the frontline, so it's not surprising that they are more prone to scrapes and damage than any other feature. Many signs of damage can be fixed, however.

Broken nail

Clip it short and clip the rest of your nails to match. There is no other way around it, other than to use one of those nail plasters that don't work very well, or to visit a salon, but who has the time and inclination to be so Princess and The Pea-like? Uneven length nails look odd. Admit defeat and go for a nice short shape in a dark blood red or black polish.

Ridges

These are common and if they are only superficial can be helped by using a buffer tool (available in any chemist) over the surface of the nail. Deep ridges are usually down to nail damage and will probably always appear in the same place (I have one on one finger where I picked away my cuticle as a child). To even things out temporarily, start with a basecoat of ridge filler. Most good nail brands do one.

Nail biting

Bitten nails are grim and you need to stop. There are nasty-tasting preventative treatments on the market but I find the most effective way to stop is to either get acrylic tips put on in a salon or, better still, gel polish. This sets so hard that nail biting is nigh on impossible and besides, your nails will look so great it will break your heart to nibble them away.

Splits

This can either be down to permanent nail damage (in which case you'll need to keep nails short and use ridge filler before painting) or more often due to very dry nails and cuticles. Use nail oil every night before bed (keeping it next to your bed will seem like less bother), massaging it thoroughly into the cuticles and nail beds.

Peeling / flaking

This is usually a result of very dry nails. Use nail oil twice a day and make sure you apply rich hand cream after every hand wash and whenever you're outside in cold weather. Gloves will also make a difference. You should see an improvement in 2–3 weeks.

Rough cuticles

Oil, oil, oil. I absolutely don't believe in cutting cuticles. It's painful and leaves the nail bed exposed to infection. Some manicurists do this for a clean visual result, but you will pay for it later. If your cuticles are rough, slather them in oil before bathing, then push them back gently with an orange stick, available everywhere.

Weakness / bendiness

Buy a strengthening nail treatment with calcium. These are available all over and aren't expensive. Paint on before every paint job. Some are clear and can be reapplied daily, over your nail polish, though after a couple of days everything will probably peel off. You should see an improvement within the month.

Colour chipping too fast

Quality of polish is important, but in my experience the culprit is more likely to be too thick polish. Always scrape the excess colour off the brush onto the neck of the bottle. Never use a 'fast-drying' topcoat unless you really need to, as I find they cause polish to shrink and consequently chip after a day or so.

GLITTER POLISH WON'T COME OFF

Glitter can be a nightmare to remove. To get it off thoroughly, soak a cotton wool disc in acetone-based remover (available everywhere). Hold the wet disc onto your nail for ten seconds without moving it, allowing it to dissolve the polish underneath the flecks. Then sweep away, wriggling the pad as you go.

HORRIFICALLY DRY HANDS

Winter and housework are brutal on hands, but you can make a big difference pretty quickly. Before bed, apply a blob of gentle body scrub to dry hands and massage in as though you're washing them. Rinse off. Massage in lots of heel balm (the stuff for cracked heels from the chemist), then put on some cotton socks, like mittens, before bed. Repeat each night until better, using rich hand cream during the day.

NAIL ART

I am truly in awe of women who master nail art. I could look at their imaginative creations and their often extraordinarily skilled application for hours. Nails that look like cats, watermelons, burgers, or made to look tie-dyed or covered in leopard print – I'm endlessly impressed, yet rarely indulge myself, on the basis that I don't have time to fiddle so long with something that's gone in a couple of days (I'm not quite sure they're really my look either, in all honesty). Nonetheless, I do occasionally wear stick-on wraps (easy) and have been known to cover my polish in polka dots for fun (both wraps and dotting tools are very easy to use and are available at most high-street chemists and via a million online stockists). But for in-depth nail art instruction, look to Instagram and Pinterest and be prepared to lose hours of your life.

NEXT-LEVEL NAILS

Two nail treatments beyond a non-pro's capabilities.

GELS

Shellac, Gellish and OPI GelColor are all in-salon gel colour treatments for fingers and toes. They're applied in a more complex manner than traditional polish – nail surfaces are made matte and rough by filing, then several layers of different lacquers are painted on, each left to set under a UV lamp. The joy of gels is that they're super shiny and neat and last 3–4 weeks without chipping, making them perfect for holidays, weddings and so on, and they are set completely and unsmudgeably before leaving the salon. They shouldn't damage nails unless you attempt to pick off the polish (gels must be removed by soaking them in acetone and gently scraping off with an orange stick).

ACRYLICS

Acrylics are false nail tips, essentially. They're great if you like very long nails, or want to display ambitious nail art. After cutting down the natural nail tip and filing the surface of the nails, the plastic tips are stuck on with glue, then bonded onto the nail with an acrylic mixture and placed under a UV lamp to set. They're then filed and shaped and painted as normal. Like gels, they're removed by soaking in pure acetone. They're not my personal cup of tea as I like shorter nails and could never be bothered with the salon visits, but many women are devoted to them and they can look magnificent. The best acrylic salons tend to be in areas with a high Afro-Caribbean population, where practitioners are most experienced.

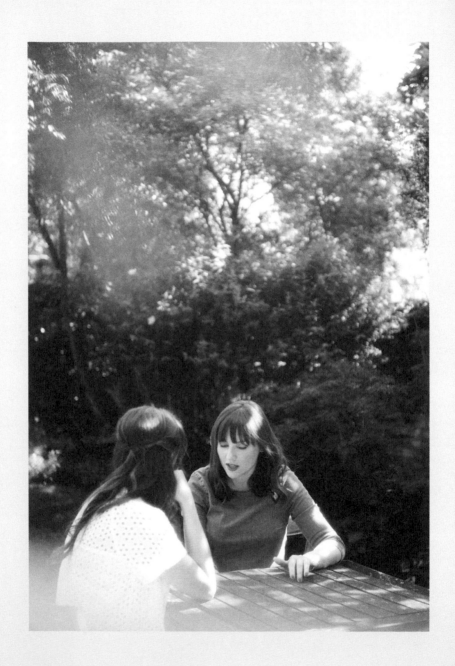

HOW TO PAY AND
RECEIVE COMPLIMENTS

*'I just think it's silly to be stingy with compliments.
If you see someone and they strike you as beautiful
in any way, why not let them know?'*
Jill Scott

At least three times a week, I stop a woman in a public place and tell her she looks fantastic. Whether I love her hair colour, or her make-up, skin or shoes, I always mean it (or else there's no point). I'm not effusive, creepy or persistent. I think the nice thing, briefly say the nice thing, then go on my way. I have honestly considered getting little cards printed with 'You look amazing' or 'I very much appreciate your look' to save time. While some women must surely think I'm a lunatic (some of them look bemused, even looking behind them for someone more obviously worthy), the overwhelming majority appear very happy to hear it. Except that after a fleeting moment's unguarded flattery, most recipients will effectively tell me I'm wrong. Her 'roots need doing', she 'actually didn't get enough sleep last night', she literally points out a zit or a coldsore with her finger, effectively saying 'No, look! You've made a terrible mistake! I'm flawed!' It makes me sad that women are so insistent on deflecting praise and believing themselves unworthy of it.

Compliments are like medicine. You may not want to take them, but ultimately, they are good for you. They are also good for the compliment payer. Sure, one of the reasons I pay compliments is because I like receiving them. I know how cheering it is when a complete stranger says 'nice tattoo' or 'I love your lipstick', especially when that stranger is a woman. There's often something more meaningful about a compliment from a member of our own team. It somehow means more – partly because we're more respecting of a woman's opinion on, say, make-up or hairstyles, but also because when a woman compliments us we can usually be sure she's not trying to score our telephone number or get us into bed. She has no motive to dish out flattery other than to be nice and because she means it.

But I mainly give compliments because making people feel good about themselves makes me feel good. They must be real to work, however – sincerity is key. People can smell token gushing a mile off, so I don't just hand out compliments like sweeties. Don't tell your friend she's lost weight unless it really appears she has (every woman knows when she's looking fat), don't say how great someone's hair looks when it resembles Friends' Monica in Barbados. Everyone has something good about them, so bide your time until you truly feel it. The art of receiving compliments is straightforward. If you're on the receiving end of flattery, please don't fight it. To reject a compliment is impolite and is potentially stopping the giver from paying another to the next person. Don't deflect a good deed, making the giver feel like they wished they'd never bothered. Just smile, say 'thank you', then take a moment to enjoy it. And next time you feel the impulse to compliment another, pay it forward.

More essential feedback

As powerful as a compliment is the sort of sisterly observation that stops other women looking crap. That doesn't mean telling someone they need to lose weight, or that their hairstyle is catastrophic, it means discreetly, kindly and swiftly giving someone the opportunity to make a quick fix before they see themselves in a mirror and want to cry. These include:

'You have lipstick on your teeth.'
This looks bad and is never anyone's intention, so quietly gesture to someone with bright red teeth that they should probably take a look. If this is also something that frequently happens to you, end every public meal with a quick glance into your knife. The reflection will alert you to the problem and you can tend to it without anyone noticing.

'You have food in your teeth.'
You must always tell someone if they have a spinach leaf or shard of pork chop stuck between their front teeth. No one wants to look like a caveman and to have everyone at the table failing to look anywhere but their food-strewn mouth. Be a good sister and let someone know.

'You have toilet paper on your shoe.'
This happens all the time in grotty public loos. Don't be THAT woman, who allows another to drag a trail of Andrex through a pub like a husky pulling a sledge. Approach someone and tell them, or be a class act by stepping on the trail so they can escape untethered.

'You have mascara smudge under your eye.'
This happens to most women towards the end of the night and it's bloody annoying. Finding yourself in the ladies room with carbon black bags, not knowing how long they've been gatecrashing your face, is grim and disappointing. Telling someone well before that moment is a great kindness.

'You have blood on the back of your skirt.'
If you do no other kindness to womankind, you absolutely must do this. Nature is occasionally cruel and a woman is caught unawares by her period. For God's sake tell her and save her from 3–6 months of feeling wholly mortified. If you're feeling extra saintly (and in this instance, it's very good karma to go the extra mile), offer her your cardi to tie round her waist.

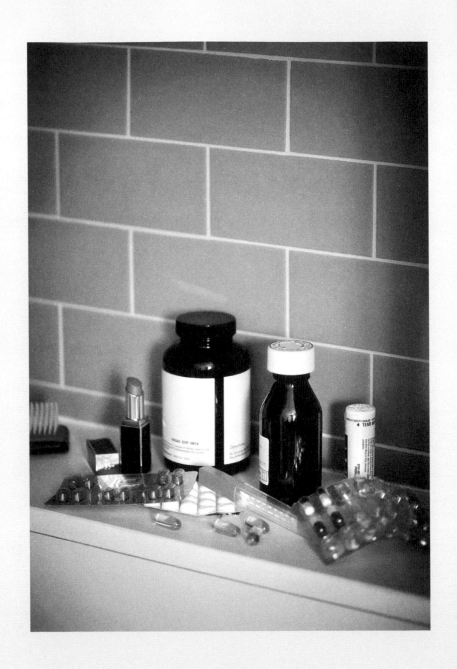

BEAUTY IN ILLNESS

'Smile. And keep putting on lipstick.'
Diane Keaton

I remember vividly being 12 and watching *Trading Places* on telly one weekend, when I suddenly yelped out and involuntarily bent double with searing kidney pain. My brothers gawped at me like a dog being shown a card trick, while my mother and Auntie Ursula, having heard the crying, came in to deal with what was probably another fist fight. After the doctor left a couple of hours later, having diagnosed a kidney infection, and people were plumping pillows, pouring Lucozade and putting on *Gregory's Girl* for me, by far the most comforted and spoiled I felt was as Ursula sat with my feet on her ample lap and painted my toenails in her Revlon Red lacquer. I felt instantly better, as much as I intended to milk a few more days off school.

A girlfriend of mine recently awoke from major surgery on a cancer in her lower leg. And what was the first thing she did, after hearing that her leg had been saved and the anaesthetic had worn off? She painted her toenails. I am endlessly inspired, though rarely surprised, by the significance beauty adopts during times of ill-health. Women with their bodies out of their hands and at the mercy of disease take control of their faces and hair. I have worked with many women in the darkest of hours, showing them where exactly to get a wig that doesn't make them look like a 1970s nana; recommending a face serum that stops people in the street adopting the dreaded side-head and telling them they 'look ever so tired', showing them a simple, short make-up routine that allows them to feel like themselves when everything else is unrecognisable.

Anyone who dismisses beauty and make-up as an irrelevance pursued by the vain not only knows nothing about women, but has zero understanding of the complex effects of illness. During the darkest times, beauty takes on an extra significance and, for many, can become one of our most effective coping mechanisms. Our appearance is so much a part of our identity. When this appearance changes through accident or ill health, there can be a process of grief and a great deal of adjustment and adaptation. Maybe your face is the least of your worries and your health means you have considerably bigger fish to fry, but the chances are that if beauty is already an important part of your life, a bout of illness is not going to change who you are.

We all know illness can be brutal on our looks, but serious illness can be especially cruel. Cancer treatment commonly causes thinning hair or baldness, skin and nail problems and weight gain or loss. For patients, the loss of one's outward identity can be a very traumatic process, and can affect their relationship with their body. In a clinical trial, 77 per cent of female cancer patients were distressed by hair loss, with many describing it as worse than losing a breast (it ranked 'worse' overall than other side effects such as nausea, insomnia and anxiety). This is unsurprising when you think that hair is arguably our most prominent physical feature and the one people very often use to describe someone –'the blonde', 'the redhead'. By 'people' I chiefly mean pillocks, but nonetheless, hair is key.

Last year my friend C was diagnosed with cancer. She had to spend several months in and out of hospital, receiving aggressive chemotherapy and lying in a bed surrounded mostly by very old ladies in their nighties. While it must have been tempting to wear pyjamas 24/7, she refused to compromise on personal grooming, putting on normal clothes each morning after showering and sitting up in bed, putting on a full face of make-up and maintaining a decent manicure and pedicure. During her stay, C confessed that in her hospital bag she had five lipsticks, three lip stains and two lip balms. I was frankly impressed by her restraint.

While our number one priority should obviously always be health, appearance is critical in how many unwell women feel day to day. With such big things happening in their lives, it's perfectly natural to me that so many women respond by wanting to feel and look as 'normal' as possible. Even the ritual of putting on make-up every day keeps a normal routine going when everything else has changed. Self-care – whether for you that means a quick shower and some lip balm, or full slap, falsies and fake tan – is very important where possible.

Over the years, I've found the issue of control also seems to be critical for many women. The ritual of applying make-up, the dignity in maintaining a pride in one's appearance, can also be a way of reclaiming your own body from cancer and the medical profession. In a 1997 study, 70 per cent of female cancer patients indicated that feeling some sense of control over a changing appearance in the context of cancer treatment was 'extremely important'. My friend C recently told me, 'People – kind, skilled, expert people – are constantly discussing and doing things to my body, and sometimes I think they forget it's mine. Painting my toenails reminds me my legs are still there and they belong to me. It irritated me recently when doctors told me off for wearing nail polish with my cast, because they wanted to inspect my toenails for signs of poor circulation. No way am I hobbling around barefoot with no nail polish. I have my limits.' I knew exactly what she meant.

For many patients, make-up is also a way to blend in at a time when physical manifestations of cancer treatment are seen as an invasion of their privacy. While no one has any reason to be ashamed of their cancer, they have every right not to be defined by it either. No one should be forced to declare their illness every time they nip out for a paper, any more than they should have to announce anything else about their private life. Make-up during serious illness is often not about being noticed, but about being ignored. Women want others to see that they are the same person as before, and for that, often the only solution is to paint on healthy.

Painting on Healthy – The Essential Products to Help to Fake You Better

Hyaluronic-rich face serum

Chemo and other strong medications often dehydrate your skin, leaving behind fine, crepey lines, flakiness and a dull grey pallor. A hyaluronic serum (applied after cleansing) will grab onto water in your skin and plump it up, as well as help brighten your whole skin colour. Clarins, Vichy, Eucerin and Chanel all do brilliant ones, but anything containing a high percentage of hyaluronic acid (a harmless, natural substance already found in healthy cells, that won't irritate your sensitised skin) will do it.

TINTED MOISTURISER

A good tinted moisturiser is your best friend when ill. It moisturises skin that will be dryer than usual, gives back a healthy glow to sallowed complexions and usually protects against the sun, making it an ideal product for when you are too weak or simply can't be arsed with the faff of multiple products. Don't be tempted by BB creams. In my experience they look lousy on skin that's not in good health. The best tinted moisturisers are by Laura Mercier, Becca, Origins, Nivea, Nars and Bobbi Brown.

CONCEALER

Everyone needs a good concealer, but never more so than when unwell. A good, dense creamy cover-up will conceal scar redness, dark circles from under- or oversleeping and spots from hormonal medications. Choose one with light reflectors to restore some glow while it hides the crap. I love concealers by Nars, Clinique, Bobbi Brown, Clarins, Charlotte Tilbury and Liz Earle.

BLUSHER

This will make the biggest difference to ailing skin. Take a perky (but not ickle-girl sugary) pink shade in a creme formulation (healthier and more natural looking than powder blush) and, using your middle finger, dab a little on the fat parts of your cheeks (if your cheeks have lost volume while ill, do an inane-looking smile to make them pop out). Blend outwards with your fingertip in a dabbing motion, until there's a circle with no clear lines. The best creme blushes are by Liz Earle, Bourjois, Tarte, Chantecaille, Becca, Benefit, Body Shop and Bobbi Brown.

BROWN EYELINER PENCIL

If you've lost your brows and lashes, this is an essential. Circling the eyes in soft smudgy brown gives them back their depth and definition and is more natural-looking than false lashes, which can look odd without the real thing as a base. Use the same pencil to fill in your brows in short, feathery strokes. If you look like Ming the Merciless, treat yourself to some brow stencils – they're fast and idiot-proof. My favourite pencils are by Elizabeth Arden, Rimmel, Urban Decay, Charlotte Tilbury and Bourjois. The easiest stencils are from Shavata Brows.

LIPSTICK

If you don't normally wear it, use a balm instead, but if you do, for God's sake, keep on. The day I give up my lipstick is the day I die. Fine to look ill if that's how you feel. Fine to slouch, wig-off and spotty into a box of Krispy Kremes if that's what you fancy, but if today's a day for faking good health, nothing will make you look more like yourself. Treat yourself to a spendy one – it's the least you deserve. Try Chanel, Estée Lauder, Nars, Bobbi Brown or Tom Ford.

SUPER-MOISTURISING FACE MASK

Illness usually involves dehydrated skin and a tedious amount of lying around doing nothing, so a face mask was made for it. Once a week, smear your thoroughly cleansed skin with a thick layer of mask. Put your feet up for 20 minutes, then either remove or massage in, according to the packet instructions. Look out for hydrating ingredients like hyaluronic acid and glycerin and gentle natural moisturisers like rose oil. Avoid anything containing AHAs and BHAs until you're better, to avoid any irritated flare-ups. Some of the best are by Clarins, Body Shop, Fresh, Kiehl's, Lush, Clinique and Origins.

A MICELLAR LOTION

This is a liquid cleanser used loads by professional make-up artists backstage at shows. During illness it's heroic. The joy of micellar is that it cleans skin thoroughly without running water, making it ideal for hospital stays or long bouts in bed. It's much gentler and more thorough than cleansing wipes (which just move the crud around your face) and leaves skin completely clean without a nasty residue, ready for skincare. My favourites are by Avène (perfect if your skin has become super-sensitive), La Roche-Posay, Garnier, L'Oréal Paris, and Bioderma. All pretty cheap. You'll need cotton wool discs too. The best and cheapest are from the Boots baby department.

A RIDICULOUSLY TREATY BATH CREME

Any illness requires some self-awarded decadence to make it bearable. Bath creme or oil is ideal, since you'll have more time to spend soaking. Choose something softening and moisturising (honey is always good, as is almond oil – neither irritates inflamed skin, unless you have a nut allergy) and don't be stingy on portions. This is not the time to be sensible. When ill, I always reach for Laura Mercier Honey Bath, or Elemis Milk Bath, which is excellent on anyone unable to take a lot of fragrance in skincare.

BUYING A WIG

If you've lost your hair and want some back, then you will need to get a wig. Here's how to do it convincingly.

CHOOSE A STOCKIST

Often the best wig stockists are in locations with a large Jewish or ethnic population. There, you are more likely to find experts who sell realistic-looking wigs to thousands of women. Large department stores like Harrods and Selfridges also have excellent wig departments, selling fashionable styles and offering expert advice. Make an off-peak weekday appointment so you can really take your time trying on lots of different wigs. Customers are often asked to pay a deposit for a proper wig appointment, but this is redeemable against a wig purchase and worth it for proper service.

KNOW WHAT YOU WANT

Whether you want something identical to your real hair, or decide to experiment with something new, be firm about what you want and how much you want to care for it (nylon wigs are cheaper and easier to look after, but look a little less realistic, natural hair wigs are spendy, higher maintenance, but are much easier to style and look like the real deal). This is your hair and it's extremely important you feel comfortable.

Don't allow a member of staff to presume that just because you've been unwell you need what I call 'cancer apology hair' – a sort of drab, short, conservative do in suicide tan. You are ill, not 104. If you feel best with long hair, glamorous waves or peroxide blonde porn hair, then that's what you should have. This is about feeling like you. If you are understandably nervous, take a friend from whom you can hear 'you look bloody ridiculous' without crying or becoming punchy.

TAKE YOUR TIME

Expect to spend at least 45 minutes trying on wigs and take pictures on your phone of any shortlisted styles that fit well (a good wig is snug, with a firm but comfortable band). Decamp with your friend for coffee and consider the styles carefully, but remember that a shop-bought wig is only the jumping-off point – it can be styled and trimmed however you'd like.

LISTEN AND LEARN

After choosing your wig, insist that the salesperson shows you exactly how to put it on, demonstrating how to pin up remaining natural hair if you have it, buying a spare net so you can wash one. A decent wig is bloody expensive and any good stockist considers this service part and parcel of the price.

GET STYLED

Look up Trevor Sorbie's fantastic charity My New Hair and locate your nearest participating salon. Make an appointment for a new wig-styling session, asking if there is a private area for this, if that's what you'd prefer (there very often is). Take along some pictures you like (either of your old hair or something you've seen) and explain how you'd like your wig to look. Lots of things are possible – a wig stylist can add soft layers, shorten the length, even add highlights to natural-haired wigs. Make sure you get plenty of advice on how you can play around with the style at home.

People who want to help you to look better during illness

The Look Good Feel Better campaign (www.lookgoodfeelbetter.co.uk) helps women with cancer by giving them a goodie bag of quality cosmetics and delivering seminars on how to use the products to make the best of one's personal appearance. Many women say the guidance helped them regain a sense of control over their bodies and offered a chance to feel feminine, normal and more confident. Changing Faces (www.changingfaces.org.uk) is a charity set up to offer advice and support to anyone dealing with the impact of changed appearance, whether through accident or illness.

....

Trevor Sorbie's My New Hair charity (www.mynewhair.org) offers a network of top hairdressers who will advise any woman suffering from medical hair loss on wig purchase and then style it free of charge. The Give and Make-up campaign (www.giveandmakeup.com) uses beauty to offer comfort to women suffering in a different way. They accept your donations of unused beauty products and pass them on to women who are starting a new life after escaping domestic violence and other dangerous situations. It's where I send my beauty samples at the end of each season, but they are grateful for even one new pot of moisturiser.

....

Caroline's Campaign (www.carolinescampaign.co.uk), founded by TV presenter Caroline Monk, awards luxury pampering days in spas to nominated cancer patients (a recent study of 100 women with breast cancer found that those who received beauty treatments reported higher body image scores than women who had not).

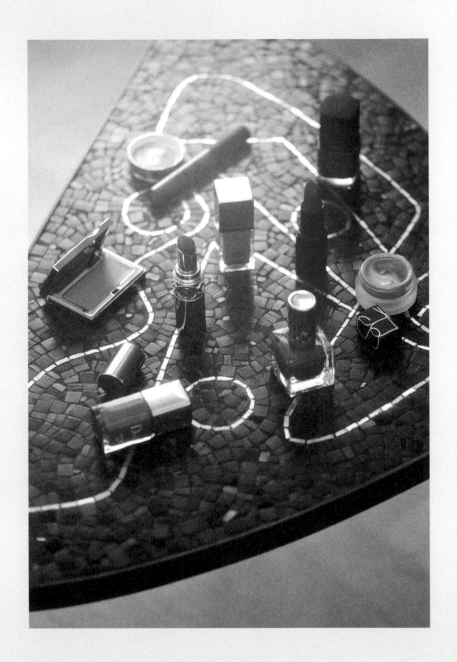

COLOUR RULES: WHO CAN WEAR WHAT?

'If you obey all the rules, you miss all the fun.'
Katharine Hepburn

For the most part, I loathe colour rules. The enemy of joy and creativity, they are usually best left to Mrs Beeton types who wash meat, salt aubergines and never wear black to weddings. I confess my heart sinks when women routinely ask me whether they can wear blue eyeshadow with blue eyes, or bronzer with pale skin, or brown eye make-up with brown and hazel eyes. Life is too short. I once had the dubious fortune of going on a cruise; one morning, I attended a 'colours workshop' out of curiosity. One by one, I watched audience members of every age and skin tone trot on stage, swathes of tatty coloured fabric held up to their faces, only for each and every one of them to be told to avoid strong colours and instead wear some joyless variation on diluted cappuccino. What balls.

In general, I think you should wear whatever shade makes you happy (if you try on a new colour that suits you, you will smile when you see your reflection. If you try to talk yourself into it, it's probably wrong for you), with only a few extremely unflattering exceptions. And yet I am all for using colour to exaggerate features you like. The truth is, some shades just look amazing on some colourings; others have natural bedmates that together create the prettiest looks. Some colours make grey eyes look vivid green, or cause ordinary blue eyes to pop and sparkle; while others get rid of ashiness in black skin, sickliness in pale. A mismatched manicure and pedicure is essential, while a mismatched lip and cheek looks like you're an extra in a Robert Palmer video. Confused? Here are the few self-designed rules by which I for the most part abide.

Don't: Wear pink eyeshadow if you're Caucasian.
With almost no exceptions, pink eyeshadow, from pastel to cerise, makes white women look like lab mice. What's more, the lighter shades make everyone of any skin tone look old-fashioned and mumsy. Pink eyeshadow is simply not sexy, unless it is a very uncompromising shade of hot pink worn on women of colour (pale pink can make dark skin look ashy) – then it is a bold fashion statement. It works in no other context.

Don't: Wear peach or purple lipstick if you're a smoker.
Unless you get your teeth whitened regularly, peach or purple lipstick is a bad idea. Both make teeth appear even yellower. If you want to wear lipsticks in the same general ballparks, swap peach for bright coral or reddish orange, and substitute purple for berry and rose tones. Even if your teeth are gleaming white, frosted or glittery peach lipstick is truly the end of days. Stick to matte or creme finishes.

Don't: Wear pinks and blues together.
This is practically the only colour combination that unfailingly horrifies me. There's something very 'little girl raids her mother's make-up bag' about it. It's sickly, a bit cheap and immature-looking. If you wear pink lipstick and like cool eye tones, opt for slate or charcoal grey. If you're hooked on blue shadow, wear it with coral, brown, caramel or peach lips.

Don't: Be afraid to wear shadow in the same colour family as your eyes.
Conventional wisdom dictates that blue eyeshadow should never be worn on blue eyes, brown shadows on brown eyes, and so on, lest one drowns out the other. Nonsense. All you need to ensure is that your shadow isn't exactly the same shade as your irises, which is practically never the case anyhow. For example, my eyes are pale green and dark emerald or bottle-green shades look great and make my eye colour pop. Navy and brown eyeshadows are neutrals and look good on everyone, the former giving your face a smart and chic elegance, the latter, an earthy depth.

Don't: Wear dark shades of lipstick on very thin lips.
This is just one of life's little screw-overs and anyone on the receiving end has my sympathies. Dark lipstick makes very thin lips look even thinner and will almost certainly bleed. Instead, opt for paler lipsticks or, if you want a flash of colour, wear it in a sheer gloss finish. Neither will shrink an already small mouth.

Don't: Attempt to darken your face with foundation.
The job of foundation is to mimic your natural skin. You can warm it slightly with a yellow-toned base, but attempting to darken it with a mismatched foundation will look grubby and false. I completely understand the occasional impulse to look a less deathly shade of white, and positively share it, but this is the task of bronzer and blusher, layered over your base.

Don't: Wear mismatched cheeks and lips.
One of blusher's primary roles is to ease the journey from lips to eyes, not jar in the middle. I am not saying you need to painstakingly colour match your blusher and lipstick (though if you feel like it, or want to wear one product as both, this looks absolutely fine), but I am saying that staying within the same general colour family for both lips and cheeks is the most flattering and modern way to go. For example, I always wear peach, coral or apricot lipstick with a blusher in any one of the same shades. With pink, rose or red lips I wear blusher with a pink undertone. Stripes of orangey blush worn with pinks and reds looks very eighties and a bit naff.

Don't: Avoid wearing black and navy together.
Ugh. People who quack on about black not matching navy are idiots and are missing out on truly one of the chicest combinations there is, in both fashion and beauty. Navy shadow with black liner is completely gorgeous, even necessary (black is the only liner that can hold its own against very dark shades) and gives the sexy Parisienne look that I adore.

Don't: Skip red because your teeth aren't perfect.
If your teeth are slightly yellow you can absolutely still wear red. You just need a bluey base rather than an orange one to brighten the entire mouth and provide strong contrast with your teeth. See the chapter on Red Lipstick for more advice.

Don't: Wear pink-toned foundations.
Unless the palest yellow shades are still too dark (as is the case in no more than about 5 per cent of women), then avoid reddish (Afro-Caribbean) and pinky (Asian and caucasian) foundations. They just don't look nice and leave a sort of waxy, sickly finish to all other skin tones. A shade with the word 'rose', 'rosé' or 'blush' in the name is usually one to avoid.

Don't: Think purple is only for other people.
Purple is a very broad church and there's a shade within it for everyone. If you look bad in violet (dark-skinned girls tend to look awesome in it, anyone paler needs balls of steel and a huge personality to carry it off), then branch out to softer shades. Super-pale girls look good in greyish heather and soft mauve, while Asian and Afro-Caribbean skin tones can look absolutely beautiful in aubergine and garnet shades (I'm unkeen on plum, especially since it seems to be the default recommendation for dark skins by people who can't be bothered to learn what actually works). Lilac should be banned on everyone over nine.

Don't: Think you have to wear brown mascara if you're blonde.

Blonde women who grew up reading magazines have been convinced in large numbers to wear brown mascara for fear of looking 'harsh'. This is nonsense. Yes, absolutely brown mascara can look very pretty and natural on lighter-haired women (I particularly love it on anyone when worn on the bottom lash, while traditional black coats the top. If you can be bothered with the faff, it looks fantastic), but black suits everyone, including blondes and redheads, and gives a defined, glamorous finish. And unlike brown, it comes in countless formulations. Which reminds me...

Don't: Wear coloured mascara on its own.

People who say coloured mascara is naff are miserable and plain wrong. I own mascaras in navy blue, emerald green, metallic bronze, rich aubergine, graphite grey – even silver. I use them to add interest when I don't feel like a big eyeshadow look, or as a nod to an item of clothing I'm wearing, or just because they're fun. I never apply them alone, however. They are, to me, a finishing touch, an accessory, not mascara as such. Use classic black for definition, thickness and glamour, top and bottom, then stroke one coat of colour over the top, either on the upper lashes only, or on both decks. Either looks fabulous.

Don't: Decide you have to have pale brows to match your pale hair.

Watch a Hitchcock film and you will see that there are few things more chic than a blonde with dark brows (see also: Sharon Stone, Madonna and Naomi Watts). Plenty of redheads and blondes have naturally dark brows and lashes, and so my feeling is that if nature is not consistent on these matters, then make-up certainly needn't be. Tint brows dark if you feel like it, or keep them pale and darken them with pencil or powder as and when it takes your fancy.

Don't: Wear pastel eyeshadows with strong-coloured clothes other than black.

I am not generally a fan of pastels on grown women, unless they are worn with dark eyeliner (pastels like pistachio and powder blue go well with chocolate brown) and with either pale or black clothes. Conversely, clothes in strong colours like red, hot pink, orange, yellow, purple and cobalt blue look bloody awful with pastel make-up because they get to sort of trample all over your face and shout it into submission. You immediately go into the background, looking a bit unwell, while a piece of cloth takes the spotlight. A bold lipstick, dark liner and lots of black mascara will allow your face to hold its own.

Don't: Be too matchy matchy.

Red dress worn with hot pink lipstick isn't just okay, it's preferable. Ditto pink dress with bold orange or red lips. A well-chosen clash adds some interest, looks more modern and stops you looking like you've spent weeks planning a fancy outfit. It's less pedestrian, more insouciant and knowing to clash a little. I extend the theory to fingers and toes – mine are never matching. Who wants one colour when you can have two?

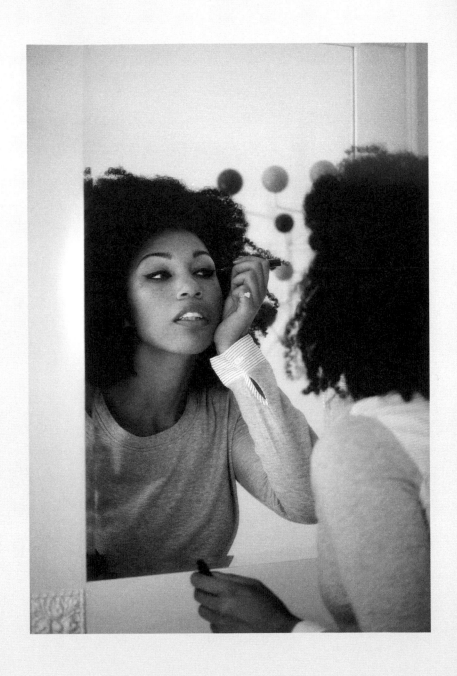

SOME THINGS YOU THINK ARE HARD – BUT AREN'T

'Make up is very, very easy.
It's only us that makes it difficult.'
Val Garland

I have very shaky hands and can barely draw, but since I was around six years old I've always approached make-up as a series of fun puzzles to solve. Black winged eyeliner seems harder than hell, but it's not. You just need to know you should use a pencil under the liquid to banish all slipperiness. Covering a huge spot seems impossible, but it's not. Can't do a bun? You need an old sock, pronto. I have amassed a lifetime of beauty tricks that make the hard stuff a cinch – even in the hands of a beauty novice. Here are just a few.

WINGED EYELINER

Those iconic feline flicks of liquid eyeliner, beloved by Bardot, Monroe, Fonteyn and so many other glamorous women, will never go out of style. I wore flicky 60s liner for years and while it will always be a look I love, I've parked it momentarily until its huge moment in fashion passes. Because the point for me is that flicks are special – they require effort, patience, maintenance, occasion and a half-decent outfit. I don't want to wear them when everyone's at it. There are still times, though, where only a flick will do and I'm terribly grateful for my ability to draw them.

The flick is really not that hard to do if you treat it like riding a bike – it's like adding stabilisers and then removing them when you're feeling more confident. The stabilisers come in the form of a black pencil. Its marks will be completely covered, but it is just tacky enough to stop the liquid-liner brush wobbling and veering off course.

Start by lining your eyes normally with the black pencil – going from the inner corner towards the outer. Stop when you get three-quarters of the way across your lid. Then, using the same pencil, make a tiny dot wherever you'd like your flicks to end. I generally imagine the corner of my eye to be either 3 or 9 o'clock, then place my dot 5–10 minutes further towards 12 o'clock. Put the pencil down and swap it for a liquid eyeliner pen or separate brush dipped in liner gel. Using the tip of the pen, join the dot with the tail of your pencil liner. Sweep it across the pencil line. Allow to dry with eyes closed or looking down, then adjust any differences between the two eyes if necessary. Finish with mascara. Over time, you will become dexterous enough with the liquid liner to stop using the pencil. But there's no hurry.

NB: This look doesn't work especially well on very wrinkled eyelids, or on hooded ones. Don't sweat it. There are heaps of other make-up looks you can try.

A BALLERINA BUN

There's really no need to buy one of those cheap, nylon, clip-in buns you see on infomercials. Just get an old odd sock and cut off the foot so you have a long-ish tube. Put your hair in a ponytail, its base wherever you want your bun, and secure with a hair elastic. Pull the ponytail through the sock tube so its length is encased. Now, starting with the end of the sock at the tip of the ponytail, roll the sock back, outwards (as though removing a stocking), smoothing your hair over the top of the sock to conceal it as you go. Tuck any loose hairs under the bun. When you can no longer see any sock, secure with a couple of grips across the bun's foundations.

DEFINING THE SOCKET LINE

People drive themselves round the bend applying eyeshadow, but it really is much simpler than you think. If you can put in a darker crease line then, frankly, the job is pretty much done. A darkened crease makes lids look more defined, larger, more colourful. The trick is to go slightly above the natural socket line, not in it, otherwise any colour will just disappear as soon as you open your eyes. After applying a neutral base colour all over the lid (ivory works on everyone), take a small, domed, natural-haired brush (I hate to play favourites but the best ever is MAC's 219 – I have at least six of them) and coat it well in a slightly darker shade. This can be taupe, bronze, mushroom, khaki – anything, in fact, as long as it's darker than your base colour and paler than your liner. Dab the brush on the back of your hand to remove excess powder and then, with your elbow resting on the table, pivot your hand like a windscreen wiper from the outer end of the socket line to the inside, a couple of millimetres above the natural line. Always start on the outside as this is where you'll want to deposit the most shadow, getting fainter as you approach the middle. That's it.

CLUMP-FREE MASCARA

I'll admit to sort-of liking clumpy mascara on occasion, but for everyday lashes you want them darkened and thickened, but separated. The key is always to dab the point at the end of your mascara wand onto a tissue or the side of the tube before applying. Otherwise the blobby bit, if left on, just moves around the lashes causing clumps. When your wand is de-blobbed, look down into a mirror and lift up your eyelid with your thumb if necessary. Take the wand from root to tip, wiggling from left to right as you go. The wiggling movement deposits maximum colour without clumping. After applying one coat, switch eyes and re-load your wand, repeating the process. Then go back to the first eye to apply a second coat in the same way. When the wand is almost empty of mascara, use the same wiggly motion on your bottom lashes.

CONTOURING

At the time of writing, the world has gone completely mad for contouring. YouTube and Instagram tutorials abound, presented by far more committed and gifted contourers than me. Do look them up; they're soothing to the point of hypnotic – Charlotte Tilbury and the Pixiwoo sisters are all lovely and expert make-up artists with a very nice and reassuring manner. Personally speaking, though, I feel the moment you decide you don't like your natural face shape, you are headed down a path of high-maintenance grooming that will suck the lifeblood from your mornings – and I skip breakfast for no cheekbone. However, I completely understand the impulse to sculpt the face a little, so here are the basics.

Contouring is made up of highlighting and lowlighting. Lowlighting uses a darker colour than your natural skin to recede anything you'd like to slim or make less prominent. For this you'll need a cream concealer or stick foundation (MAC, Iman, Inglot, Laura Mercier, theatrical brands and Illamasqua all make great ones) in a colour some three or four shades darker than your skin. The texture here is important because you need to be able to be precise and stick to one area at a time without the colour bleeding elsewhere. By contrast, highlighting uses a lighter shade than your natural skin tone to accentuate areas and bring them to the fore. For this, a matte or very lightly shimmery cream a few shades lighter than your natural skin tone is best. Pearly highlighter is fine on pale faces, but it looks frosty and space-age on dark skin, so a bronzy highlighter is best with any natural skin tone darker than olive. You will also need a small round brush that can be buffed into the skin. I like MAC Duo Fibre brushes (a mix of synthetic and natural hairs) best.

When you have gathered together everything you need and you've applied your foundation, coat the brush with your dark cream and suck in your cheeks. Draw a diagonal line in the hollow then, using downward buffing strokes, blend the dark cream all down the sides of the face beneath the hollow, being careful to stay at the sides and not wade into chin territory. You can use the same technique on your temples if you like. Blend and buff thoroughly – there should be no streaking nor brush marks. The highlighting part comes next and is easy. Take your paler cream and, using your middle fingertip, dab it onto your cheekbones, above the dark shade in your hollows. This will thin the cheeks but emphasise their bones. Set with powder.

APPLYING FALSE EYELASHES

False eyelashes have become hugely popular in recent years, and yet, still many women imagine them to be near impossible to apply. I feel the same way about falsies as I do about tying a bow tie – they're only worn occasionally but it is a satisfying skill to have up your sleeve. There are two golden rules: you must always cut strip lashes to size first, trimming them from the outside end in. A lash strip that's even a tiny bit too long will bump up against the bridge of your nose and peel off (probably before you've even left the house). The second is to never attempt to apply lashes when the glue is wet. This makes them slip, wobble and peel. What you need is an almost dry, tacky finish, like when you got Pritt Stick on your fingers as a child. If the lashes fit and the glue is tacky, the lashes will go on and stay there.

COVERING A SPOT

Covering a spot is highly satisfying when you know how. See the Bridal chapter for a full how-to.

A NOTE ON BRUSHES

Good-quality brushes are 100 per cent worth the cash. They make everything easier and neater. I find the mistake that women make most often with eye make-up is that they try to do the brush's work for it, overriding its natural stroke by moving their arms about when usually only a pivot of the wrist is necessary. The shapes of the bristles, the brushes' materials and handle shapes, their weight and length, are all chosen according to their job. Don't think you know better and muscle in – just hold the brush and go with it. My brush collection includes many different brands (like hi-fi equipment, brushes are best bought individually, no one brand is the best for every type of brush), but wherever you choose to shop, you will need the following:

1. A fat powder eyeshadow brush, about 1.5cm wide. I like natural bristles or a mix of natural and synthetic. The edge of the bristles should be rounded. This is for laying down base colour and for blending colours together to soften edges.

2. A smaller powder eyeshadow brush, about 1cm wide. Choose natural bristles and a rounded shape. This is for laying down colour on the lids.

3. A crease (or 'pencil brush'), a small, slender, short, natural-bristled brush with a bullet-shaped tapered tip. This serves several purposes, including adding definition to the eye crease, softening hard liner and adding smokiness beneath the eye. The best example is a MAC 219 – I strongly suggest you invest.

4. A fat powder brush with a rounded bristle. This is for applying a very light coating of face powder or bronzer, or for removing excess powder after applying with a puff. It's also extremely useful for blending way-over-zealous blusher or bronzer application – just dip it in fine translucent powder first. Your powder brush needn't be very expensive because it's doing a pretty imprecise job, but I still recommend you choose one with a domed bristle-head rather than one that's cut across like Louise Brooks' fringe.

5. A chubby blusher brush. Most of the blusher brushes I see are way, way too small. A good blusher brush is quite chubby and rounded (this is why brushes in blush compacts are the absolute pits and need to be binned immediately). The bristles should be natural and domed, with a nice solid handle for good control.

6. A concealer brush. I never apply concealer without one. You just get a much more precise, opaque coverage with a brush versus your fingertips. I personally like my concealer brush to be duo-fibred and quite small. The MAC 286 is my concealer brush of choice, but many prefer a flat lip-brush-style for applying cover-up. Each to her own.

7. A mascara spooly. This is essentially a clean mascara wand on a brush handle, but you can wash an old mascara if you can't be bothered to buy one. In any case, budget and brand are, broadly speaking, unimportant.

Optional
Foundation brush (I use one for better coverage than fingertips), a lip brush (I never use one, ever), a separate bronzer brush, a liner brush (depending entirely on whether you use gels, pencils or liquids with brush applicators), synthetic or duo-fibred brushes for applying cream shadow or blush (I use these but you can easily skip them and use fingertips), a synthetic, stubby, angled brow brush (I'm never without one, but what can I say? Brows are my thing).

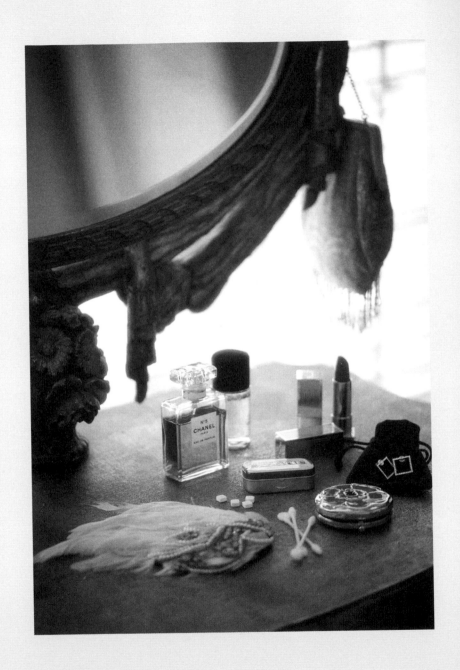

BRIDAL

'It is beautiful to be what you are.'
Jean Paul Gaultier

I adore weddings and consider it a great honour to have been able to design the make-up for so many of them. It's a joy to work with a bride on one of the happiest days of her life and thrilling to see the photographs afterwards and see that I helped her to look as good as she felt.

That said, I find bridal beauty a bit of a weird concept. To me, it is really just special occasion make-up – albeit the *most* special of all occasions – and should be treated accordingly. A bride should look like herself on the best day ever. Her usual skin tone should be at its most flawless, her go-to special hairstyle at its most perfect, her signature going-out make-up at its most immaculate. A man or woman is marrying you, so it has never been more appropriate and, frankly, polite that you try to look like you, the person they fell in love with.

That is why I am perpetually stunned at how many brides walk down the aisle looking like someone else. Ringlets on straightening-iron devotees, fake tan on pale skins, sickly pastels on those rarely seen without bold lips and dark, sultry eyes. Padded bras on flatties, elaborate fake hairpieces on short hair. Enough! A wedding day is not the time to play at being a flaxen-haired virgin from a Disney fairytale. It's a time to look like you at your most amazing.

Not that I'm suggesting you whack on your everyday make-up as though between bus stops en route to a breakfast meeting. There are special considerations. Your everyday make-up only has to look good until you take it off. Wedding make-up needs to still look great in 30, 40, 50 years' time. An ordinary night out doesn't involve hundreds, sometimes thousands, of photographs being taken, or being stared at by an entire crowd of guests. Bridal make-up needs to be long lasting, immaculate, showstopping and future-proof.

So how do you get it? Women, in growing numbers, are booking a professional make-up artist for their big day and it can be a very wise investment. But, for reasons that remain unclear to me (perhaps in some misguided attempt at avoiding a busman's holiday), I booked a top celebrity make-up artist for my wedding and I honestly rue the day I picked up the phone. She was brilliant, unflappable, talented and kind, but that is not the point. She didn't know me. She applied soft pink lip gloss when my rose bouquet and visible lining of my dress was lipstick red, my signature colour. She expertly blended warm, earthy brown eyeshadows over my lids, not knowing that I would still be looking at them 13 years later and thinking how they jarred against a cool-silver vintage silk dress. My brows were nude, not sculpted as I like them. I looked fresh-faced when I am all about the good base. My small eyes looked smaller. I basically had a perfect face of make-up that I'd never have allowed on anyone else. Learn from my mistake.

A professional – either a freelance make-up artist, beautician or beauty counter artist – can be a great idea if you lack the skills, calm and dexterity to do a great job yourself. Very often, though, a skilled and honest friend can be just as effective (I normally offer my services to friends by way of a wedding gift), though you must never accept the offer if you're even remotely unconfident in his/her abilities – you only have one shot at this and you don't need the stress of a bad make-up job.

Whether hiring a pro or calling in a favour, a pre-wedding trial is absolutely essential. This is where you can play with different looks, talk through your personal style and preference, iron out any problems, test the skin for any reactions, leaving the day itself completely free and calm to just apply what you already know looks great. They should take place a good month or so before the wedding, but after details like dress and flowers have been nailed down. Book your trial on a day you have nice evening plans. I so hate to see good make-up go to waste.

On the day, you will need to allow one hour for make-up, 45 minutes for hair. You may well not use anything like as much time, but this allowance will guarantee minimum stress. Plan everything you need in terms of product, and group your kit together in a transparent case or bag (if you've hired a pro, they should already have done this). Wash your brushes in advance and take a picture of your trial face if you need reminding. Make sure your bridesmaids are properly briefed if they're doing their own faces – you don't need the hassle of worrying about them. Wear your dressing gown or PJs for the makeover, but apply lips last, when dressed and otherwise ready. Don't try out anything new; go with what you know looks good, what you know you or your pro can do well, and what makes you feel absolutely bloody amazing.

Bridal treatments

Some appointments worth making:

2–3 facials
Get one a month (if you can afford) for the three months running up to the wedding. Make the last one a couple of days beforehand. I don't recommend having your first and only facial very close to the big day in case of any reaction to new products, make it the week before.

Gel manicure
These month-long paint jobs are brilliant for weddings and should last you through your honeymoon too. They give a plump, super-shiny finish that looks perfect in close-up pictures and won't chip or smudge for a few weeks. Gels also reduce the chance of a last-minute breakage, as they make the nails super-hard. They must be removed by soaking in acetone – do not be tempted to pick or you'll ruin your nails.

Professional blow dry
Pay a hairdresser to come to your home/hotel, or make an early salon appointment for the wedding morning. It will be the best £30–60 you spend. If you wear your hair down, wash it without conditioner and get them to give you the kind of amazing blow dry you'd love to have every morning. If you often wear your hair up, check that your stylist is experienced in up-dos. Do not get curls where there are none, nor try to go straight when you normally wear waves. If you have Afro hair, get an Afro stylist, if you have European hair … You get the idea.

Lash extensions
If you are all about the lashes, these can be a great wedding investment. Synthetic lashes are glued onto your own to lengthen and thicken them. They remove the need for mascara, making them perfect for criers, and look wonderful in pictures if applied properly. They're expensive (from £50–150) but should last until the end of your honeymoon.

Wedding emergencies

Shit happens. Here's what to do in a beauty crisis.

Crisis: Tan lines
Many brides fail to protect their skin in the run-up to their summer weddings and end up with white bra-strap lines. If this happens to you, you need a body foundation cream or wash-off tan to fill in the white gaps.
Solution
Choose a darker shade of body foundation (Mac and Fake Bake make great ones) than your skin, to match with the dark patches.

Apply to clean, unmoisturised skin (body lotion will cause streaking and clothes staining), stroke the foundation over the white patches, blending outwards over the lines. Allow to dry for a few moments and repeat if necessary.

Dust loose powder over the area with a fat, fluffy brush. Leave for a few minutes before getting dressed. Drape a clean napkin, scarf or tea towel over the neckline of your dress as you step into it.

Crisis: Coldsore
Coldsores suck so hard and I pray for you that they leave your wedding well alone. Here's the best you can do if not:
Solution
I cannot recommend enough the Boots Avert coldsore machine, which has changed my life for the better. If you are prone, get one now and treat yourself twice a week, whether a sore is brewing or not. If you are unlucky enough to feel a sore coming close to your big day, zap it every couple of hours with the machine.

At night, apply coldsore patches to stop reinfection and spread via pillowcases. Remove them as soon as you get up and continue with the machine and cream, if desired.

If the sore is still obvious and has yet to scab over, see a private doctor or dermatologist as soon as you can and get a cortisone shot to reduce redness, pain and swelling. It is worth the money.

Wear a clean, new coldsore patch on the day. These can be covered with make-up and mean you can kiss your loved ones without fear of infection. Change the patch regularly.

Tell your photographer that you would like the sore and patch retouched out of any close-up pictures. This is easy for any decent photographer to do.

Crisis: Spot

In very extreme circumstances, i.e. when there's a zit the size of a family saloon on your chin, make an emergency appointment at a private skin clinic and ask for a shot of cortisone into the area. The spot will heal very quickly. For smaller, less ruinous, spots, here's what to do.

Solution

Take an antihistamine. Cleanse your face thoroughly and use a BHA-based liquid exfoliant. Moisturise with an oil-free moisturiser or a face oil designed for oily/combination skin.

If you have time the night before, make an aspirin face mask for the affected area only. Crush five aspirin tablets with a rolling pin and mix into one tablespoon of full fat natural yoghurt and one tablespoon of honey (skip the yoghurt if you have dairy allergies). Massage over your face. Leave on for 10–15 minutes before removing with a hand-hot flannel. Follow with an oil-free moisturiser. Obviously avoid if you are allergic to aspirin. I don't believe at all that this mask will get rid of your spot, but it should reduce redness and swelling.

On the day, apply some brightening eye drops directly to the clean spot area. Wait a few minutes.

Apply primer and foundation, patting lightly over the spot.

You are now going to make my Hughes Club Sandwich. Tap a little matte concealer cream (not a highlighting pen) over the spot, feathering outwards.

Dust with loose powder.

Repeat the previous steps until spot is completely covered. Always finish with the powder layer.

Crisis: Uneven self-tan

I cannot stress enough that your wedding is not the day to try new things. If you are not proficient at self-tanning, or if everyone is used to seeing you looking very pale, then don't go there. But if you or a salon has applied self-tan badly, resulting in orange elbows, knees and feet, here's how to help sort it.

Solution

As soon as possible after dodgy application, apply rich body moisturiser and massage it into your entire body, using circular motions. This dilutes the active tanning ingredient making mistakes far less obvious. Pile on the cream here – the more generous, the better.

Get a couple of fresh lemons and cut in half. Rub two all over the streaky areas and don't rinse off. If your elbows are bright orange, place the remaining two lemon halves sliced-side up onto the table and rest your elbows inside them. Stay there for 15–20 minutes.

Even out any remaining patchiness with body make-up (see Tan lines, above).

Crisis: Runny eye make-up

There's usually a fair bit of crying done at weddings. Here's how to safeguard your make-up in the event of emotional displays.

Solution

Always wear a primer under your wedding make-up. This will help it go on smoothly and stay there. Strong eye make-up will require a separate eye primer to stop liner transferring onto the lids. Many brands now make them. Tap them on with your ring finger after your foundation, before eye make-up.

Even if you think you won't cry, it's essential you wear a waterproof mascara, or a waterproof sealant over a normal mascara. Alternatively, you can get lash extensions, lash tinting or wear falsies and forget mascara altogether.

Always make sure someone in the wedding party is carrying cotton buds and non-oily eye make-up remover, to make any unexpected clean-ups throughout the day.

Never, ever use any product for the first time on your wedding day. If you are a little bit allergic, your eyes will stream.

Do not 'cleanse' with wipes the night before (I am absolutely convinced these cause many women's eyes to stream the following day). Use a proper cleanser and remove it with a hot cloth.

Get an early night. Tiredness causes watery eyes.

Enjoy a glass of wine or champagne with your friends on the eve of your wedding, by all means. But don't drink more if you want your skin to look its best in the morning.

Bridal bag essentials

You need these with you on the day. Dump them on your bridesmaid or mum if you're not carrying a bag.

Lipstick
I don't care how much you're enjoying yourself, please, please, please keep an eye on your lipstick. You will be eating, drinking and kissing all day and even the most skilled make-up artist won't be able to apply lipstick to withstand that. If you let it wear off, you will regret it when the photos arrive (trust me, I've been making up brides for 20 years. I've seen it happen over and over). Touching-up lipstick is a two-second job once every couple of hours. Keep on top of it.

Mints
It's a very long day and Champagne has an unfortunate effect on breath. Some sugar-free mints (not gum – it looks terrible with a wedding dress. See also: alcopops) will keep you feeling fresh.

Powder compact
Pressed powder is the fastest, easiest way to keep make-up looking perfect over the course of a long day. Every couple of hours or before photographs, press the lightly coated puff into any shine (usually on the chin and nose) using a rolling motion.

Perfume
I wouldn't go anywhere without perfume – least of all my own wedding. Buy a tiny travel atomiser like Travalo and fill with your favourite scent. Spray after the wedding breakfast (strong perfume when people are trying to eat is not nice) and before the evening reception, to freshen up.

Cotton buds / Q-tips and travel bottle of non-oily make-up remover
These are absolutely essential for cleaning up smudges, mascara run, kiss prints on your face, any mishaps down your dress (oil-free eye make-up remover is the best stain treatment). They may seem a faff to carry, but when you need them, having them to hand is a godsend.

Glasses
It may sound obvious, but if you need specs to apply make-up, you'll need someone to bring them if you're not wearing them. So many brides forget this amid the fuss.

Six bridal looks that look great

The best bridal looks are the ones that look most like you, but in my experience, there's something below for every personal style. Over the past two decades, I've had a great deal of success with these bridal looks, chiefly because they're flattering, feminine, look timeless and don't date your wedding album.

1. Vintage movie star
Face
Flawless base, gold eyeshadow, black flicky liner, arched brows, red lipstick, black mascara and pinky-peach cheeks.
Hair
Glamorous waves, sexy up-do.
Suitable for
All skin tones, all ages.

2. Gamine ballerina
Face
Fresh, glowy base, taupe smoky eyes, soft brows, black winged liner, pink, nude or red lips.
Hair
Short or a sleek, simple up-do like a chignon or bun.
Suitable for
All skin tones, all ages.

3. Sixties sex kitten
Face
Matte base, smoky eyes, lash extensions, pale pink cheeks, lined matte lips in nudes and pinks.
Hair
Backcombed, tousled bed hair, either down or up in a modern beehive (avoid going too high or it'll look like fancy dress).

All skin tones, those under 35.

4. Soft and romantic

Face

Dewy base, earth-toned eyes in browns, berry and plum, dusky rose blush and lipstick.

Hair

Soft, casual waves or curls.

Suitable for

All skin tones, though the darker the skin, the less dusky the rose tones should be – opt for a brighter rose, berry or pink. All ages.

5. Bronzed and sexy

Face

Luminous base, earthy brown and golden shadows and liner, peach or brown cheeks, golden highlighter, glossy nude lips.

Hair

Casual, relaxed and sexy, down or up.

Suitable for

Olive to black skins, all ages – though older skins should cut down on any shimmer as it can accentuate crepey-ness in the skin. Also suitable for pale girls but err towards golden rather than very bronzed.

6. Fresh and pretty

Face

Light, dewy skin, nude-toned shadows, light bronzer, pink or peachy cheeks with matching lips, natural brows, a little highlighter along cheekbones.

Hair

Any.

Suitable for

All skin tones, all ages.

A NOTE ON SAME-SEX WEDDINGS

Two faces of make-up, rather than one, does require some planning. Again, it's important for each of the brides to look like herself, but in the interest of good pictures I'd suggest opting for two make-up looks that are complementary, but never matching. Fresh and pretty with soft and romantic, bronzed and sexy with Hollywood movie star, 60s with gamine, for example, can work very well. Two completely different looks can look incoherent or like fancy dress.

A NOTE ON BRIDESMAIDS

I really do think that, for the most part, bridesmaids' make-up should be from the same colour palette. It just seems daft for them to be wearing the same dress, colour or fabric while sporting clashing make-up. It looks messy. Choosing one colour palette – navy and nude, for example, black and red; mauves, pinks and purples – then letting your bridesmaids wear the shades in their own individual way makes for a smart and coherent look on the day. I never make-up little girls unless they especially want it, in which case I apply a little tinted lip balm and pretty creme blush and leave it at that. Don't let your little flower girls get pageant queeny, it looks creepy and weird.

THINGS TO AVOID

I'm not a big fan of beauty rules, but there are some bridal no-nos on which I stand firm.

Excessive use of light-reflecting concealer pens
They cause glare in flash photography and cause brides to suffer reverse-panda eyes. Very illuminating creams do the same. Use sparingly.

Hot trends

Your look needs to be timeless so that your pictures look great forever. A classic or even a retro look that's withstood the test of time. This is not the time to be trying something very 'now'.

Ringlety tendrils

Hassidic-style tendrils, hot-tonged to within an inch of their lives and flanking a tight up-do style. This looks completely mad on everyone and is perilously close to wedding dresses worn with Bo-Peep bonnets and a crook. No, no, no.

Not enough make-up

Weddings are unusual in that they're part special occasion, part photoshoot. It may seem out of your comfort zone, but a little more make-up than usual will look better in both. You will need primer, foundation, concealer and powder, eyeshadow, liner, mascara, brow powder, lip liner, lipstick, bronzer and blush in order to go the distance. This may seem like a lot, but if chosen and applied well it won't seem too much in photos, I promise.

Very glossy lips

Everyone will be kissing you. A jammy mouth will blur, smudge and fade. Opt for proper lipstick in a satin finish and follow my application technique in Red Lipstick.

Pink eyeshadow

It's always surprising to me that so many brides choose pink shadow, as though one must be ultra girlie as a bride. It's a mistake that makes most of us look like lab mice.

French manicure

We must never wear a French manicure. I personally love dark nails to match bold floral bouquets and set off sparkly rings, but if you'd like pastels, opt for ballet pink, taupe or apricot and paint all over the nail.

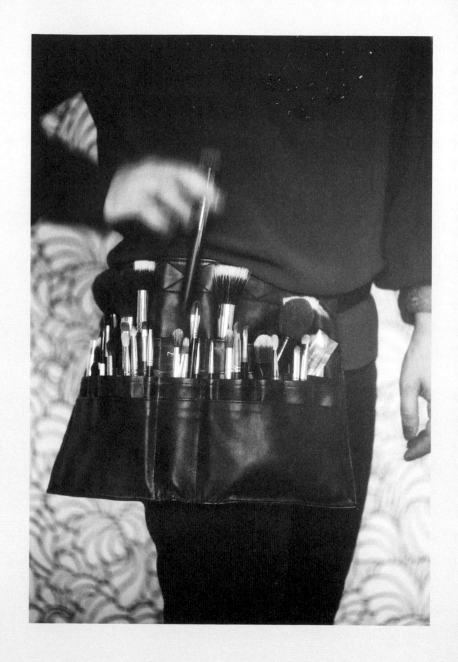

SPECIALIST SHOPS

'Ugh. Everything in department stores is pink.'
Lynne Easton

I was 15 or 16 the first time I entered a professional beauty store. I was assisting make-up artist Lynne Easton on the Pet Shop Boys' 'Was It Worth It?' video and my mission was to buy over 20 pairs of false eyelashes for the drag queens cast as dancers, who were to be dressed as my idol, Elizabeth Taylor. In those days, falsies weren't anything like they are today. Boots sold only a couple of styles, both subtle and boring. We needed huge, fancy lashes and our production budget was wee, which apparently meant only one thing: a pro store. I wasn't prepared for the sheer, giddy, joy waiting for me behind the door of Screenface in West London. Pretty paintbox lipstick palettes, imported yellow-toned foundations (such a rarity in those days) and cover-everything concealers sat on cluttered shelves next to fake blood, bruise kits, bald caps and moustache-stiffening wax. I must've stayed for two hours, playing with stippling sponges, grey stubble filings and strange brushes I hadn't yet got the faintest idea what to do with.

Over two decades later, I'm still hooked on pro stores. If I'm between meetings with an hour to kill, off I head to a pro shop or beauty salon supply store (there's one in every city) and browse the aisles, buying hairgrips by the hundreds, old-fashioned curler pins no one else seems to sell any more, hot wax pots and waxing strips that save fortunes on salon visits, fantastic unbranded pencils and powders at a quarter of the price of their department store counterparts, empty palettes to fill with old eyeshadows begging to be prised from cracked packaging and given a new lease of life. So much of my work kit – including the Zuca case it's stored in – comes from a pro store.

But you don't have to be a beauty industry worker to enjoy pro stores, you just need to love products and not be easily intimidated by shopping with professionals. In my experience, pro store staff are friendly, knowledgeable and eager to translate that to a non-professional customer. I beg you to visit. These stores need our support and contain gems you'll never find anywhere else.

Independent chemists are wonderful, too, and are invariably the first place I seek out in an unfamiliar town or village. Here you'll find lovely Bronnley soaps shaped like lemons and limes, proper Yardley toiletries, fluffy powder puffs, Mason Pearson hairbrushes (try one –

you'll never go back), travel cases for medication that make brilliant palettes for scraping old lipsticks into, Max Factor face powder and the Revlon Flex haircare you thought had vanished for good. Put me in an indie pharmacy and I'm as happy as a clam for over an hour until the staff have clearly decided I'm a bit weird and I leave £30 worse off.

Never visit foreign climes without making time for a drugstore visit. There is nothing more exciting for a product fan than aisles of unfamiliar, foreign beauty bargains. I have never once visited America without setting aside at least two hours to visit the local drugstore or beauty supply. In New York, I hit Duane Reade (for Neutrogena make-up, Cover Girl, EOS and a raft of others) and Ricky's of Broadway (for Magic Move hair cream, kitsch accessories, neon liners and wipe-clean bags). Anywhere stateside, I visit Walgreens or Target for acres of brilliant shampoos, hand soaps, dermatologist-designed skincare sold at a steal. In France, I head straight to a pharmacy for mid-price skincare from amazing brands like Nuxe, Phytologie, La Roche Posay, Bioderma and Klorane (no one does affordable but serious better than the French), before heading to Make Up For Ever for the widest range of palettes, and brushes anywhere. I may be nerdier than most, but I urge you to at the very least add a Sephora to your holiday itinerary.

And whatever your skin tone and hair type, please do not ignore ethnic beauty supply stores. While the nature of their business can't and shouldn't be classed as specialist, their broadly independent status makes them so. As high street brands are slowly, and rightly, becoming more inclusive and online stores sell anything you can think of, I fear that ethnic beauty shops will lose their younger customers. This would be a terrible shame if allowed to gather pace, because these stores are packed with fantastic products you just don't see anywhere else. Huge vats of divine scented cocoa butter for a couple of quid, top-quality combs and hair tools, better and cheaper nail supplies than anywhere on the high street, wonderful coconut, almond and wheatgerm oils and rich, skin-softening shea butter, bargain treats from fantastic old American brands like Queen Helene and Dax. These places are goldmines for beauty fans. As with all professional artistry shops and salon supply stores, it really is a case of use them now or lose them later.

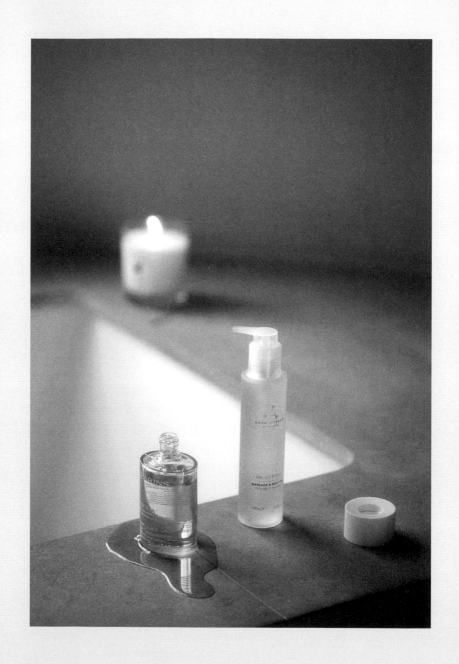

SAVING THE BEST FOR NOW

'Always use the good bath oil.'
Nora Ephron

My heroine Nora Ephron often said that the death of her best friend had taught her one thing: to always use the good bath oil. This sums up exactly how I feel about beauty. I'll explain. One Christmas about ten years ago, Crème de la Mer sent me the most exquisite gift box containing a fortune's worth of lovely products. It was so pretty, so luxurious, so perfect, that I put it in the cupboard to keep safe. I resumed my normal skincare routine, thinking that one day, when I was feeling very special, I would open the box and become briefly the kind of woman who slathers on Crème de la Mer just to pick out a wheely bin from B&Q.

So there the box stayed for the next four years, except when it moved house from a cupboard in London to a cupboard in Brighton. One day, as I got ready for a posh wedding and felt decidedly frumpy in that post-partum way (see Beauty and Motherhood on how to deal with this), I decided that the Crème de la Mer would be just the thing to make me feel better. Out the box came and as soon as I unscrewed the lid of the first lovely ceramic jar, so did the smell. Everything had gone off and was fit only for the dustbin.

This, I realised, was a metaphor for life, and never again would I make the same mistake. Too many women think that maybe one day they'll go blonde, or spritz the gorgeous perfume, or open the luxury body cream, or light the spendy candle a friend gave them. We use the crap china, saving the wedding-list crockery for some imaginary 'best'. We keep the lovely cashmere jumper that makes us feel sexy and beautiful hidden away in mothballs where it can give us no pleasure, choosing instead to wear the unflattering old T-shirt on the school run. Our mums did it, their mums and grandmothers did the same before them – all unconsciously but very clearly saying that we don't deserve lovely things now, that they are for another, more refined woman, or a time when we can justify treating ourselves. What utter balls we women will believe in order to keep ourselves down.

Saving things for best is like metaphorically spending your life sitting on a sofa wrapped in cellophane, waiting for a more deserving time that may or may not ever come. And even if it does, the sofa will be out of fashion, the perfume will have soured and be fit for nothing but stripping pine. And besides, any opened serums and creams should be used daily or at least weekly in order to work, so using them only on special occasions is a big old waste of cash. We are not rehearsing here. We are alive now and deserve to look and feel great. Buy the neon lipstick, pour the luxury bath foam with abandon, light the candle for no discernible reason and wear the Chanel No5 to the Co-op. Lovely things deserve to be seen, used and enjoyed, not hidden away. And you deserve to live well and feel great now, not later. Life is really bloody short, so stop saving things for best today. It really is a mug's game.

How long things keep

Most products have a shelf life that is marked clearly on the box with a picture of a jar and a time frame, for example '18m'. This means that, once open, you have this long to use it before it either goes off or the ingredients become inactive. As for the rest...

Brow gel

Buy cheap (brow gel is only hair gel in a mascara wand) and throw it out every six weeks. There is no way of keeping brow gel clean – it picks up loose make-up particles and goes cloudy and gross.

Mascara

People say you should chuck mascara every six weeks, but if you are using it every day and only on yourself, it will last until it's finished. If you are an infrequent user, then throw it out after about four months. In any case, you will stop your mascara from drying out if you twist the wand, not ram it in and out like a bicycle pump. The same applies to liquid liner. Before you throw away a mascara, bear in mind that a clean wand is very useful for de-clumping lashes and grooming brows, so wash it in a non-moisturising shampoo and leave to air dry on a clean towel.

POWDER EYESHADOWS AND BLUSHERS

Powders last for ages and ages. I have eyeshadow palettes in my kit that I bought when I was 16 and they still blend perfectly with no irritation. If anything powdery has a film of ick on its surface, looking gross and stopping brushes from picking up colour, take a blunt butter knife and gently scrape it off, revealing fresh make-up underneath.

CREAMS AND LOTIONS

Anything liquid or a cream has a distinctive smell when it's gone off, but in fact it may have become ineffective long before that. Follow the use-by guidelines on the box. Unopened, you generally have around two years to use them up, but I would obviously suggest using and enjoying them now. Life is short.

NAIL POLISH

Nail polishes can separate and split over time, or if kept in a warm atmosphere. Shake the bottle vigorously to re-amalgamate. If this works, you're fine to keep using it. If not, it's time to say goodbye. Keep your nail polishes somewhere cool; a fridge is not necessary, as much as I know many people do this; frankly, the space could better be used for cheese and wasting it on beauty products makes you seem like one of those tragic women who only has vodka and nail polish in. If your polish becomes claggy, drop in a tiny amount of acetone-based remover and shake well. This will act as a thinner and may rejuvenate it.

LIPSTICK

Some lipsticks last for years, others start to smell or adopt a sort of granulated consistency that looks and feels horrible. Keep infrequently used lipsticks in a cool environment and throw away if the consistency or smell changes. If you are particularly attached to a discontinued colour, slice off the end of the bullet and see if that helps (lots of bacteria lives on the exposed surface).

LIP GLOSS

Lip gloss in itself is not a huge problem, but the wands get really smelly if used infrequently (the same applies to concealers that have a wand or brush applicator). The soft tip picks up bacteria from the mouth, which then breed inside the tube. If this happens, I'm afraid the only way is out. Bin it immediately.

FOUNDATION

Open foundation lasts around 8-10 months if you shake before applying and close the bottle properly after each use. If your foundation changes colour, then it has become oxidised and needs to go. If it has separated within a reasonable lifespan, you may well be fine if you shake it vigorously. Dry bits of foundation around the mouth of the bottle are not a problem and can be used as a makeshift concealer in extremis.

CONCEALER PENS

These clickable pens of light-reflecting concealer last a long time as the product is protected inside the tube, but the brushes must be washed frequently to stop the spread of bacteria-causing spots and under-eye reactions (this is pretty common and does not mean you are allergic to the product itself). They also start to smell pretty bad. After every few uses, wash under a running tap with a non-moisturising shampoo and leave to dry with the lid off.

PERFUME

Light is the enemy of scent. Keeping perfume on a windowsill will kill it faster than a sledgehammer. Store your perfumes away from light, ideally in their box (I don't do this myself as the bottles give me too much pleasure). Metal canisters give the greatest longevity (like Armani's She and YSL's Rive Gauche), but a glass bottle of great-quality perfume could last up to ten years if stored properly. If your perfume has drastically changed smell or colour, then I'm afraid it's curtains.

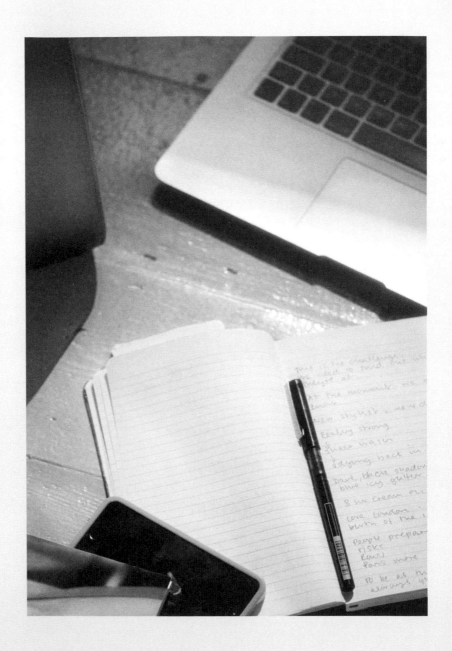

BEAUTY RESOURCES: WHERE TO GET REAL ADVICE

'The critic is the only independent source
of information. The rest is advertising.'
Pauline Kael

I am obsessed with magazines and would even go so far as to say I owe my career and love of beauty to the late, great *Just Seventeen*. I love magazines even more than I love newspapers –and I have learnt a vast amount from reading and working on mags – but when it comes to beauty coverage, it's important to explain what we're dealing with. All glossies must give positive beauty coverage to their advertisers (usually the mega corporations like Estée Lauder, Chanel and L'Oréal). If there's space left after those brands have been covered, the beauty editor can then make her own choices from the vast number of products on the market. Glossy beauty editors, though many of them brilliant, super-knowledgeable and willing, simply cannot be wholly honest (much as they'd like to be) about products in print. However, this is not the case in most, though not all, newspapers.

We are all savvy enough to live with this, I think, provided there is some balance. This is where bloggers can offer another way. Broadly free of the shackles of advertisers, they can – and mostly do – offer more honest coverage. Sometimes they are experts, but even the countless bloggers who aren't still provide a valuable discourse in a somewhat homogenous industry. For me, magazines are about great ideas, expertise, unrivalled access and beautiful, inspiring shoots. Blogs are about honest, inclusive coverage with the freedom to speak to more diverse readerships, which is both enviable and vital. (Women of colour, for example, are far, far better served by the internet than they are by print media in Britain, which basically ignores them.) Newspapers perhaps offer something between the two. I'd hate to be without any of them, though, and people need to stop pitching one against the others as though one is inherently superior or worthwhile. There are a number of resources across all three platforms that I'd like to share – magazines that have the most inspiring photoshoots and beauty ideas, blogs that cut the bullshit, forums populated with real beauty nerds, and writers with integrity. This is a list of those that I refer to most in daily life, but it is no substitute for getting stuck in yourself and finding the one you love. There are literally millions of beauty tutorials and blogs online, countless great magazines on the shelves (buy them or they will definitely go for good). My list is by no means exhaustive, is entirely personal/subjective and absolutely nothing should be inferred from omission.

CAROLINE HIRONS

Caroline Hirons is a qualified beauty therapist, beauty brand consultant, blogger and friend of mine who has particular expertise in skincare. She and I don't always agree and we very much like it that way (we enjoy a scrap over toner), but whatever our disagreements, I respect her enormously. She can be trusted. Her blog (www.carolinehirons.com) is excellent – updated regularly, funny and honest, helpful and informative. She will often reply to friendly readers' queries. Her tone is reassuringly strict and no nonsense, but kind.

LUCA TURIN AND TANIA SANCHEZ

It is probably extremely unpolitic to recommend someone else's beauty book here, but I cannot write about perfume without mentioning Luca Turin and Tania Sanchez's, *Perfumes: The A–Z Guide* (Profile). This is not only my favourite book about perfume, but is also, I'm pretty sure, my favourite book about anything. I will be thrilled if I inspire in you even the slightest intrigue about perfume but if I do, please make this your next purchase to learn from the best. No one writes about perfume like these two and no one makes the act of smelling scent sound quite so exciting and joyful.

KATIE PUCKRIK

I first met Katie when I was fifteen; she was a dancer for the Pet Shop Boys and I was first make-up assistant for their videos. I stayed in beauty, she became a DJ and TV presenter who developed an enormous crush on perfume. She now writes an excellent and entertaining blog on scent which includes fragrance reviews and videos. Find her at www.katiepuckriksmells.com.

INDIA KNIGHT

India is the much-loved beauty columnist on *Sunday Times* Style. She is sort of the anti-beauty editor, in that she rarely knows what's new, doesn't attend launches and seminars and doesn't really regard herself as an expert at all. What she is, though, is a discerning 40-something woman who gets absolutely giddy about good products and treatments, and she has good taste. She is wholly independent, fiercely honest and passionate about what she likes, and is great fun to read.

PIXIWOO

Two make-up-artist sisters, Sam and Nic Chapman, who host a hugely popular series of real and achievable tutorials on YouTube. Apart from being very good make-up artists, they have a skill for conveying information warmly, unpretentiously and inclusively. They are very, very nice women, which makes the whole thing a cosy way to spend a few hours.

KATE SHAPLAND

Kate Shapland is the beauty editor at the *Telegraph* Magazine and has been a senior and extremely well-respected beauty journalist for very many years. She is passionate about beauty and a huge supporter of small brands without the advertising budget required to secure glossy magazine coverage. She is trustworthy, independent, talented and incorruptible. She has her own business, MyShowcase.com, which brings niche beauty brands to a house-party setting.

ALESSANDRA STEINHERR

Alex Steinherr is a glossy beauty editor working under the same restrictions as all the others, but for me she is remarkable because she absolutely knows her business and is clearly consumed by it. Her passion and expertise are visible on the pages of UK *Glamour*, where she is Beauty Director, despite there still being a necessary tick-box approach to advertisers.

I am also a keen reader of Nicola Moulton at *Vogue*, Annabel Meggeson at *Red* and freelancer Jan Masters, amongst several other great beauty editors too numerous to mention.

JO FAIRLEY AND SARAH STACEY

Two very well-regarded former beauty editors now at the helm of the excellent Beauty Bible series of books. These are based around unbiased product reviews from a large panel of normal women of varying ages, colours and skin types. Products are graded honestly and clearly to help you shop. Jo also has her own perfume blog (www. thescentcritic.com) which is excellent.

ROJA DOVE

If you ever have the chance to attend an in-store perfume appreciation workshop with Roja Dove – grab it with both hands. This is the man who first inspired me to learn about perfume. His knowledge is unrivalled, his passion is infectious. He owns his own Haute Parfumerie in London's Harrods and makes frequent guest appearances at department stores and boutiques around the world.

A MODEL RECOMMENDS

Ruth Crilly, a successful model of many years' standing, blogs and presents on her own site (www.amodelrecommends.com), talking about beauty and fashion from behind the velvet rope. Like Pixiwoo, she is warm and likeable and frequently partners up with other influential bloggers like Caroline Hirons.

MAKEUP ALLEY

A vast internet community where members all over the world contribute reviews of practically every beauty product known to woman. Short reviews are accompanied by a score out of five, with average scores posted for each product. An extremely useful resource to anyone thinking of trying a new product.

ALLURE.COM

Ask any beauty junkie which magazine she loves most and she'll say *Allure*. This American magazine is the gold standard in terms of beauty coverage. It has the classic formula of good lifestyle writing: serious about silly things and silly about serious things; and carries a huge amount of authority in its entertaining, stylish, tongue-in-cheek prose. Here you'll find hundreds of reviews (albeit written with advertisers in mind), meaty features on scientific breakthroughs, great interviews with beauty insiders and excellent tutorials. The photography is beautiful too. The new interactive iPad subscription is one of the best of its kind.

SALIHUGHESBEAUTY.COM

Naturally I'm going to recommend my own site, but I specifically urge any beauty nerd looking for kindred spirits to explore the forum, where thousands of like-minded women congregate every day to talk honestly about beauty, children, relationships, clothes, books and politics. You'll also find thousands of first-hand product reviews – there's always someone who's tried a product, usually several. Also home to my 'In The Bathroom With...' series of interviews, which you may enjoy if you're as nosey as I am.

VAL GARLAND

Probably the most creative make-up artist in the world, Val Garland's online insight into her world is endlessly inspiring. Follow her on Instagram and Twitter for backstage photographs, tips, and honest, unbiased product endorsements under her 'VALidated' banner.

THANDIEKAY.COM

A beauty website launched by BAFTA-winning actress Thandie Newton and world-renowned make-up artist Kay Montano, to promote inclusive beauty across all ages and skin colours. Including tutorials, personal anecdotes and reviews, it has a very positive, woman-centred approach and is especially useful as a gateway to other blogs – many of the writers here have really good blogs of their own which often contain good writing and great advice for women of colour.

PAULA BEGOUN

Nicknamed the Cosmetics Cop, American author Paula Begoun has sold 2.5 million beauty books, mostly with a skincare theme, and now sits at the helm of her own product empire. She is mainly concerned with identifying what she perceives to be effective, helpful or harmful ingredients and has a comprehensive online database of her findings. She is not a scientist or a dermatologist, but a committed researcher and self-taught beauty expert. She speaks a lot of sense. Her large following (many of whom contribute on her community forum) is devoted to her. I am not (possibly because she thinks blue eyeshadow should be banned), but I am nonetheless very glad she exists in an industry that needs more like her.

CHARLOTTE TILBURY

Charlotte is one the world's most sought-after make-up artists and has worked on campaigns for every big name from Tom Ford to Chanel. She specialises in very glamorous, sexy make-up, which she demonstrates regularly on her own blog, charlottetilbury.com. She uses a variety of products in her videos, but also has her own (very brilliant) make-up range which is available at Selfridges and Net-A-Porter.com. She's also great value on Instagram as @CTilburyMakeup.

SAM McKNIGHT

For decades now, Scottish hairdresser Sam McKnight has been the photo session stylist, working on everyone from Kate Moss and Cara Delevingne, to Madonna and Princess Diana. He has a brilliantly entertaining Instagram account (@SamMcKnight), where he posts great fly-on-the-wall snaps of his uber-glam life in the beauty industry as well as strangely soothing shots of his flower garden.

INTO THE GLOSS

An American online beauty magazine (www.intothegloss.com) with a great site and Instagram feed (@IntoTheGloss). Here you'll find fun and cleverly conceived beauty features, quirky ideas, interesting news stories and advertiser-friendly, but nonetheless entertaining, reviews.

MARY GREENWELL

If, like me, you're a sucker for the supermodel era of big hair and glamorous make-up, you'll probably already know that Mary was one the key players. She personally inspired me to join the industry, and remains one of the world's best make-up artists, with a big focus on beauty and red carpet. I love her Instagram and Twitter (@ marygreenwell) for keeping an eye on her frankly perfect looks for Cate Blanchett, Uma Thurman, Jessica Chastain and others.

STYLIST

The *Stylist* (www.stylist.co.uk) beauty department is headed up by Joanna McGarry, an extremely good beauty director with a talent for both styling and writing. Her award-winning beauty section contains interesting long-form beauty stories alongside more traditional shopping pages and product recommendations.

FRAGRANTICA.COM

A vast online community of perfume enthusiasts, with several useful functions and honest product reviews by those with a real passion for scent. One can easily pop on to look up one fragrance, only to emerge three hours later with quite a shopping list.

BASENOTES.COM

A huge database of perfumes which are searchable by ingredients, genre, house and perfumer. A very useful resource if you, say, realise you have a thing for iris in scent and want to find perfumes with that ingredient in common.

I am forever indebted to Georgia Garrett, my incredibly clever and wise agent at RCW. Enormous thanks also to Louise Haines, Georgia Mason and everyone at Fourth Estate, and Sam Wolfson, Steph Stevens, Louise Brown, Virginia Norris and Jane Shepherdson, all of whom so completely understood this book from the off and were so utterly skilful and professional throughout. Extra special thank you to the inimitable Mary Greenwell, a childhood heroine who somehow manages to be even more clever and fabulous now, in real life.

Great love and thanks to my family: Wyn and David Hughes, Jake Walters, Sarah Morgan, Julia Marcus, Richard Wormwell, Paul Simper, Jason Burns, Victoria Reynard and Rachel James, who was one of the recipients of a Clinique soap dish when we were 11 years old and is still indulging my obsession 28 years later by agreeing to be photographed for this book.

I feel extremely fortunate to have the women of the salihughesbeauty. com community behind me, always asking questions, pushing my knowledge, telling me when something's either completely life-changing or totally crap. Do join – these are the women you wish you'd gone to school with. Thank you to all of them, and the moderators, and especially to my co-founder Debra Brock, assistant Lauren Oakey, columnist Michael Hogan and the amazing community admins who've so brilliantly held the fort during the writing of this book and who make me cry laughing every day – Fi Nightingale and Nicola Ridings Watson.

A very special thanks in particular to India Knight, Sam Baker, Nat Saunders and Lucy Mangan. Four very dear friends who have been so endlessly supportive, generous and encouraging of me and of this book and whose suggestions are always useful and wise. Thanks also to all the incredible beauty PRs upon whose dedication and efficiency I rely so heavily (you are insanely good at your jobs), and to my day-job editors at *Grazia, Red, Guardian Weekend* and *Glamour* for their support and tolerance during the completion of *Pretty Honest*. And of course, heartfelt thanks to the incomparable Daniel Maier, whose total belief in me expressed through relentless nagging in a wide array of loud and annoying voices made me finally sit down to write it in the first place.

Finally and most importantly, thank you to my beloved and beautiful boys, Marvin and Arthur. I'm sorry for all the times I can't play because I have to work. Every last word I write is for you. xx

Design and Art direction
BLOK
www.blokdesign.co.uk

Photography
Jake Walters
www.jakewalters.com

Styling
Steph Stevens
With special thanks to Whistles
www.whistles.co.uk

Make-up
Mary Greenwell at Premier Hair and Make-up
Sarah Reygate at My-Management
Sali Hughes

With thanks to the Estée Lauder archives for providing the vintage compacts

Hair
Louise Brown
Ole Amodio at Hershesons

Hair, Make-up and Beauty Assistant
Lauren Oakey

Thank you to the friends and readers who kindly
agreed to appear alongside me in this book
Polly Samson, Rachel James, Claire Jamieson, Wendy Garrett,
Judy Campbell, Eva Lazarus, Jodie Moynihan, Jo Tutchener-Sharp and Sonny Sharp,
Verity and Frances Spragge.

Additional thanks to
Nicholas Pearson and Daisy Garnett, Peter and Emmanuelle Peri,
Jane and Ben Kilburn www.kilburnnightingale.com, Jane and Steven Collins. Real Patisserie,
Brighton www.realpatisserie.co.uk, Bert and May tiles, bags from Merryn Leslie,
jewellery from Karin Andreasson www.karinandreassonjewellery.com and
Juliette Collins www.geoffreyslondon.com.

Sali's Instagram: @salihughesbeauty
Twitter: @salihughes
Website: salihughesbeauty.com
#PrettyHonest

Fourth Estate
An imprint of HarperCollins*Publishers*
1 London Bridge Street
London SE1 9GF
www.4thestate.co.uk

This Fourth Estate paperback edition published 2016

First published in Great Britain in 2014 by Fourth Estate

Text copyright © Sali Hughes 2014

Photography copyright © Jake Walters

Sali Hughes asserts the moral right to be identified as the author of this work

A catalogue record for this book is available from the British Library

ISBN 978-0-00-754981-8

Set in Knockout by Hoefler and Co, and FreightText by Joshua Darden

Printed and bound in China

Permission to use the images on the Beauty Icons title page:
Christy Turlington – Getty; Elizabeth Taylor – Getty; Josephine Baker – Estate of Emil Bieber/KlausNiermann/Getty; Kim Deal – Getty; Anne-Marie Duff – John Lindquist/ Getty; Alabama Whurley – courtesy of Morgan Creek; Zadie Smith – Sebastain Kim; Coco Chanel – George Hoyningen-Huene/RDA/Getty; Barbra Streisand – Alamy; Joan Collins – Cambridge Jones/Getty; Lauren Bacall – John Stoddart/Getty; Madonna – Gary Heery.